BACK CARE BOOT CAMP™

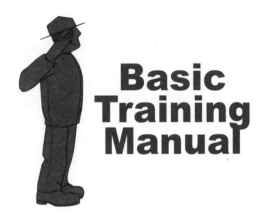

Basic Training Manual

Brent Dodge, PT, OCS, CMPT, CSCS
with
Jennifer Brooke, PT, RYT
Mary Frank, PT
Randale C. Sechrest, MD

Medical MultiMEDIA Group

Published by Medical Multimedia Group, LLC
228 West Main St., Suite D
Missoula, M 59802-4345

PUBLISHER'S NOTE
The ideas, procedures, and suggestions contained
in this manual are not intended as a substitute for
consulting with your healthcare provider.

ISBN 0-9773647-0-4

Printed in Missoula, MT
Gateway Printing

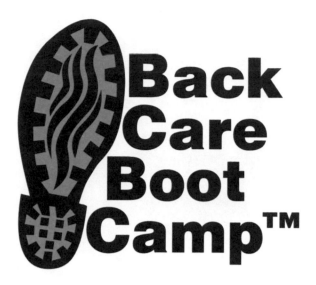

DISCLAIMER

This workbook is designed to be used during a treatment program for low back pain supervised by a healthcare provider.

The information contained in this workbook is compiled from a variety of sources. It may not be complete or timely. It does not cover all diseases, physical conditions, ailments, or treatments. This workbook does NOT take the place of working with a physical therapist or physician. This workbook should only be used in conjunction with a supervised physical therapy program. The information should NOT be used in place of an individual consultation, examination, or visit with your physician or other qualified healthcare provider. You should never disregard the advice of your physician or other qualified healthcare provider because of any information you read in this workbook. If you have any healthcare questions, please consult your physician or other qualified healthcare provider promptly. Always consult with your physician or other qualified healthcare provider before you begin any new treatment.

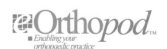

Table of Contents

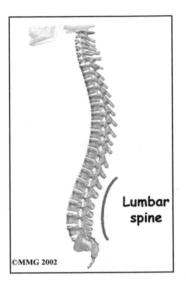

Lumbar spine

©MMG 2002

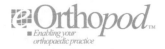

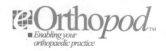

Introduction: Patients

Join the Ranks

What? *Back Care Boot Camp*? About now, you might be thinking, "Hey, I didn't join the army!" Perhaps you didn't. But the fact that you're reading this introduction probably means you've had back pain or a back injury. If so, you have joined the growing army of people who've had back problems. Experts say that as many as eight out of 10 people will have back pain that hampers work or play in their lives.

If you feel like a new recruit, don't worry. You won't be asked to hit the floor and do 20 pushups. But when you've had back pain once, there's a 90 percent chance you'll have it again sooner or later. The key is knowing how to take care of problems when they happen and how to lower your chances of future problems. That's what *Back Care Boot Camp* is all about.

A successful military effort requires planning, preparing, and responding—along with a healthy dose of discipline. Likewise, people who've had back problems do best when they have a plan, when they prepare, and when they respond using ideas and methods that work. *Back Care Boot Camp* provides the information and resources to help you succeed in this mission. We're counting on you to provide the needed discipline by applying the tips and strategies you'll learn.

Why *Back Care Boot Camp*?

The number of people afflicted by back pain continues to rise. The economic costs are staggering, but so are the costs in discomfort, pain, and suffering. Granted, most people who have back pain for the first time feel better within six to 12 weeks, regardless of the treatments they do (or don't) get.

Most people who've had back pain once don't get better by themselves. They may begin to have less pain, but that isn't always a sign that everything has returned to normal. Scientists have determined that having back pain, even once, can alter the way your back and abdominal muscles work, which can leave your spine unsupported and prone to another injury. That's where *Back Care Boot Camp* comes in. It details these new facts. It also teaches you ways to energize your muscles again to protect your back and to reduce the chances of having a future problem.

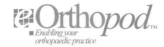

Unfortunately, a small percentage of people with back pain don't get better right away, and they end up with long-term (chronic) back pain. About 10 percent of these chronic cases account for more than 80 percent of the costs for low back pain. *Back Care Boot Camp* gives immediate guidance to help you head off potential long-term problems—before they occur.

Back Care Boot Camp is built on the most recent information. The experts who designed the program have sifted through global resources and identified the best methods and information for helping people with back pain. When you've completed the program, the syllabus and accompanying information are yours to keep. So you'll always have a handy resource that is filled with references, tips, and strategies you can use again and again.

What's in It for Me?

The *Back Care Boot Camp* program includes eight sessions that are designed for eight clinic visits. Each session is divided into seven main sections.

 Goals: Goals are listed at the beginning of each session. Read each goal carefully, and focus your energy on the most important elements of the session.

 Information to Master: Read this section in detail. It will help you understand why your therapist wants you to practice a particular skill or do a specific exercise.

 Answers for Review: Use this session to compare your answers from last session's Questions for Review.

 Skills to Master: These skills give you the nuts and bolts on how to take care of your back. Each skill includes a rationale, a description, a recommendation, and a list of possible concerns. Practice only the skills shown by your therapist. You'll be asked to demonstrate these skills at the next clinic visit.

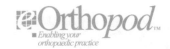
*■ Enabling your
orthopaedic practice*

Drill Time: This is your opportunity to demonstrate the skills you've been practicing. Your therapist will drill you and make sure you're doing each skill correctly.

 Questions for Review: Take a few moments to answer the questions listed in this section. They form a summary of the information and skills within the session.

 Review: The key points of the session are listed for a quick review and can be used as a refresher in the future.

Your Mission

Your mission is to learn all you can about taking care of your back. *Back Care Boot Camp* is just one resource to help you succeed in this mission. It is best used as part of a comprehensive therapy program. Always follow the advice of your doctor and therapist. When you've completed the program, you'll be a seasoned veteran who knows how to successfully take care of your spine.

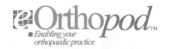

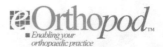

Introduction: Physical Therapists

A New Era in Back Care

Times have changed. So have the approaches used to successfully treat and manage low back pain. The challenge we face as physical therapists is to consistently provide our patients with the best treatments and information available. The task of consolidating and delivering the newest and latest research on spine care is daunting. That's where *Back Care Boot Camp* can help.

Patient education is paramount to successful outcomes when treating patients with low back pain. The key is to provide current and evidence-based information. *Back Care Boot Camp* is a compilation of global guidelines and research, so you can be sure that your patients get up-to-date information—every time.

In this new era, we often face a time crunch that limits one-on-one time with our patients. And it's our back patients that often need more of our time. We're also faced with fewer and fewer visits due to a managed-care environment. The *Back Care Boot Camp* program consolidates the information and skills we want our patients to assimilate. Implementing *Back Care Boot Camp* can help you maximize your efficiency, while ensuring that your patients get what they need.

Who Benefits?

Patients

Today's patients are hungry consumers searching for the latest and best resources and information. *Back Care Boot Camp* provides them with a unified core of knowledge.

Patients learn by doing. The course syllabus is interactive, so patients can begin to put the new information to work right away. The syllabus follows a session-by-session format, which keeps patients on track over the course of care. Your patients have continuous access to the information. And the syllabus is theirs to keep, so they'll always have a valuable resource to which they can refer.

Patients take an active part in their rehabilitation. The program minimizes passive interventions. Patients are directed to take an active role in the

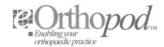

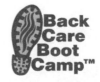

management of their spine condition. The final sessions promote active strategies for life-long spine care.

Today's literature promotes a sports-medicine model for patients with low back pain. Obviously, this enthusiastic approach must be applied only where appropriate. It should be adjusted for the aging adult, for example, who may need to proceed more slowly. In general, patients do best when encouraged early on to resume normal activity as soon as possible. The beginning sessions of *Back Care Boot Camp* help you direct your patients toward this goal.

Physical Therapists

Back Care Boot Camp is not a fixed protocol. It is a valuable tool that you can use to enhance your health-care delivery. The program is not meant as a substitute to a complete rehabilitation program. Nor is it to be used in lieu of a formal physical therapy evaluation.

Use the program to save time in the clinic. You can spend your valuable time evaluating and treating your patients. Because *Back Care Boot Camp* provides much of the information you need to relay, you won't find yourself bogged down with all the details of patient education. The syllabus supplements the information you intend to deliver.

The *Back Care Boot Camp* syllabus ensures consistent delivery of the information and skills patients need to take control of their back condition. You won't have to worry about getting interrupted and inadvertently leaving out vital information during clinic visits. You can add as much additional detail as you like during the course of care.

Back Care Boot Camp was designed using clinical guidelines. The guidelines chosen include the Agency for Health Care Research and Quality in the United States (formerly the United States Agency for Health Care Policy and Research), the Cochrane Collection Back Group in the United Kingdom, and the New Zealand Guidelines Group.

The program is outcomes-based. Track patient outcomes from start to finish using the forms included in the *Back Care Boot Care* program. You can document these changes in the *Progress Flow Chart* form, and add the form to the patient's chart. Use these records to promote your results and your approach

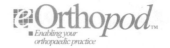

to helping patients with back pain. To avoid bias, remove the scoring forms prior to issuing patients the syllabus. These forms are located in Appendix A under "Providers."

Referring Providers

Your referring providers also benefit. When they become familiar with *Back Care Boot Camp*, they can prescribe the program with confidence—knowing what their patients will be doing and learning every step of the way. And you'll be able to communicate with your referring providers using the resources available in the program, including the outcomes measures, forms, and handouts.

Brent Dodge, PT, OCS, CMPT, CSCS

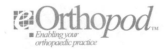

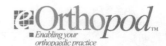

Why *Back Care Boot Camp*?

Taking care of patients with low back pain is challenging.

Most of us who have spent any significant time caring for patients afflicted with chronic low back pain realize quickly how little patients understand about their back and the problems that face them.

We all think we are great communicators, but reality tells us otherwise. Too often, we are guilty of spouting off some theory about what we think is causing the patient's pain, why we are ordering the MRI scan, why we are prescribing three or four medications, and what the patients should do to help themselves.

The problem is that we don't give patients what they really need, which is a clear understanding of how their back works and good instruction about what they can do to help themselves. Instead, we give them incomplete explanations and a pamphlet of exercises that they often don't understand. We expect them to be compliant, but we sometimes fail to give them the tools to be compliant.

We're often too busy to do the right thing.

As my frustrations grew, so did my intention to solve this problem. How could I be sure that my patients were getting off to a good start in caring for their back pain? How could I ensure that they were learning the information and skills they needed to reduce their risk of future back problems? How could I ensure that someone was taking the time to explain the anatomy and body mechanics in a way that my patients would understand? And how could I help my patients know why they were doing their exercises?

Back Care Boot Camp is the result of that frustration. I worked with three physical therapists, Brent Dodge, Mary Frank, and Jennifer Brooke, to create a core curriculum of information and skills. We felt that every back patient should have the opportunity to learn and master a specific curriculum. The result is a body of information that ensures that all patients receive the necessary tools to care for their back pain.

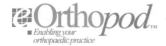

Back Care Boot Camp is the resource that most patients need.

The program is not intended to limit what the physical therapist does with the patient. We realize that each patient is unique, and a one-size-fits-all approach is not appropriate. The physical therapist is the expert in assessing the needs of the patient and providing a plan of treatment to fit those needs. But all back care patients need to understand a core of information and master a common set of tools to care for their back pain. *Back Care Boot Camp* is designed to present the core of knowledge that all back patients need to know and use.

Back Care Boot Camp accomplishes this goal through a syllabus that delivers clear, concise information to the patient. The program is not ambiguous. There are clear expectations for both the patient and the physical therapist.

Why should you use *Back Care Boot Camp*?

Back Care Boot Camp simplifies your life and improves care for your back patients.

Back Care Boot Camp provides you with the comfort of knowing that your patients will be getting a comprehensive, consistent, evidence-based approach to their back problems. When you refer your patients to a physical therapist using the *Back Care Boot Camp* approach, you know what your patients will be doing and learning.

Back Care Boot Camp improves communication among providers and ensures appropriate and timely referral and intervention.

Back pain is a complex disorder. Current research on the natural history of back pain clearly shows that the condition cannot be understood or effectively addressed by a simplistic disease model. The condition represents a multifactorial, biopsychosocial condition.

Assessment tools are built into *Back Care Boot Camp*. They are designed to provide practitioners with ample feedback for identifying associated comorbidities. They also facilitate decisions about early intervention and timely

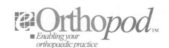

referral to specialists. You receive this information quickly, helping you communicate effectively with insurers and other third-party payers.

Back Care Boot Camp helps you translate complex information in a way your patients can understand.

Most patients who present with back pain have little knowledge of how their back works or the cause of their pain. For many, this is the first serious medical condition they have faced. We as practitioners shouldn't expect these patients to develop a satisfactory understanding of these issues in one or two visits. This is new territory for these patients! Information mustn't simply be thrown at them; it needs to be presented in a fashion that is digestible and *understandable*.

Back Care Boot Camp provides patients with information in a logical, incremental fashion. When patients understand the rationale behind a particular recommendation, they are much more likely to make the behavioral change and continue the exercise or activity. *Back Care Boot Camp* is a system designed to engage patients' cognitive abilities and senses in order to help patients sustain the behavioral changes that are necessary to improve the natural history of back pain.

Each lesson in *Back Care Boot Camp* builds on previous successes in mastering earlier material. Each lesson combines immediate physical *doing* in addition to cognitive *learning* so that each skill begins to be reinforced immediately. The multimedia tools provided in this program address all learning styles. The information is delivered in multiple modes including text, visual, auditory, and active participation.

Try the program for yourself. See if your patients benefit as much as mine have. See if it makes your life easier. I am optimistic that you'll be delighted with the results.

Randale C. Sechrest, MD
Medical Director
Montana Spine Center

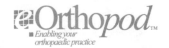

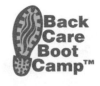

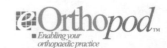

Induction

Call-Up Notice

It's time. You've gotten your call-up notice, and you've been directed to present yourself to the enlistment depot, your physical therapist's office, at the designated time. Most likely, it won't be at 0600 hours, as most therapy clinics don't open till at least 0700 hours!

Your induction marks the time when you will begin your transformation from an ordinary citizen with back problems to an active participant in *Back Care Boot Camp*. But before you jump in with both boots on, there are a couple items that you can tidy up. No, we're not talking about shining your brass belt buckle and getting the wrinkles out of the bed sheets.

Induction Papers

You've got some paper work to do, soldier. Begin by filling out the forms included in this Induction. Follow the directions carefully. Your therapist will record your answers. Unless your doctor or therapist suggest otherwise, you should proceed by filling out the following forms:

1. Patient Specific Functional Scale
2. Oswestry Disability Index
3. Visual Analog Scale
4. Fear-Avoidance Beliefs Questionnaire

Marching Orders

Now that you've gotten your call-up notice and have completed your induction papers, you need your marching orders. First, if you haven't already done so, take a few moments to read over the Patient Introduction. Get familiar with the icons that represent the sections within each of the main chapters of *Back Care Boot Camp*. Second, before your first physical therapy visit, read Session One. Be sure to cover the information and skills with your physical therapist before trying the skills listed in the Skills to Master sections. Ready, then? Ten-hut!

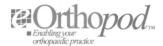

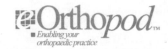

Patient Specific Functional Scale

Name: _____ Date: _____

Identify three important activities that you are unable to do or have difficulty with as a result of your problem. List each activity in the left column of the box below.

Today, how difficult is it to perform each activity?

Choose a number between zero and 10 indicating your ability to do each activity. Place your number in the score column in the box below to the right of the activity you've listed.

0	1	2	3	4	5	6	7	8	9	10

unable to
perform activity

able to perform activity
at preinjury level

	Activity	Score
1.		
2.		
3.		

Raw score _____ **Percentage (raw score/30 x 100)** _____

Source

Reprinted from *Physiotherapy Canada*. Vol. 47. Paul W. Stratford, PT, MSc, et al. Assessing Disability and Change on Individual Patients: A Report of a Patient Specific Measure. Pp. 258-263. © Stratford, 1995, reprinted with permission.

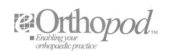

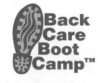

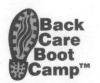

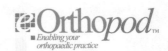

Oswestry Disability Index

Name: _____ Date: _____

The questionnaire is designed to give us information as to how your back (or leg) trouble has affected your ability to manage in everyday life. Please answer every section. Mark one box only in each section that most closely describes you today.

Section 1 - Pain Intensity

____ I have no pain at the moment.

____ The pain is very mild at the moment.

____ The pain is moderate at the moment.

____ The pain is fairly severe at the moment.

____ The pain is very severe at the moment.

____ The pain is the worst imaginable at the moment.

Section 2 - Personal Care (washing, dressing, etc.)

____ I can look after myself normally without causing extra pain.

____ I can look after myself normally but it is very painful.

____ It is painful to look after myself and I am slow and careful.

____ I need some help but manage most of my personal care.

____ I need help every day in most aspects of self care.

____ I do not get dressed, wash with difficulty and stay in bed.

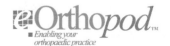

Section 3 - Lifting

____ I can lift heavy weights without extra pain.

____ I can lift heavy weights but it gives extra pain.

____ Pain prevents me from lifting heavy weights off the floor but I can manage if they are conveniently positioned, e.g. on a table.

____ Pain prevents me from lifting heavy weights but I can manage light to medium weights if they are conveniently positioned.

____ I can lift only very light weights.

____ I cannot lift or carry anything at all.

Section 4 - Walking

____ Pain does not prevent me walking any distance.

____ Pain prevents me walking more than 1 mile.

____ Pain prevents me walking more than a quarter of a mile.

____ Pain prevents me walking more than 100 yards.

____ I can only walk using a stick or crutches.

____ I am in bed most of the time and have to crawl to the toilet.

Section 5 - Sitting

____ I can sit in any chair as long as I like.

____ I can sit in my favorite chair as long as I like.

____ Pain prevents me from sitting for more than 1 hour.

____ Pain prevents me from sitting for more than half an hour.

____ Pain prevents me from sitting for more than 10 minutes.

____ Pain prevents me from sitting at all.

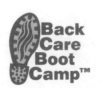

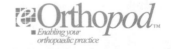

Section 6 - Standing

_____ I can stand as long as I want without extra pain.

_____ I can stand as long as I want but it gives me extra pain.

_____ Pain prevents me from standing for more than 1 hour.

_____ Pain prevents me from standing for more than half an hour.

_____ Pain prevents me from standing for more than 10 minutes.

_____ Pain prevents me from standing at all.

Section 7 - Sleeping

_____ My sleep is never disturbed by pain.

_____ My sleep is occasionally disturbed by pain.

_____ Because of pain I have less than 6 hours sleep.

_____Because of pain I have less than 4 hours sleep.

_____Because of pain I have less than 2 hours sleep.

_____ Pain prevents me from sleeping at all.

Section 8 - Sex Life (if applicable)

_____My sex life is normal and causes no extra pain.

_____My sex life is normal but causes some extra pain.

_____ My sex life is normal but is very painful.

_____My sex life is severely restricted by pain.

_____My sex life is nearly absent because of pain.

_____Pain prevents any sex life at all.

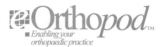

Section 9 - Social Life

____ My social life is normal and causes me no extra pain.

____ My social life is normal but increases the degree of pain.

____ Pain has no significant effect on my social life apart from limiting my more energetic interests, e.g. sport, etc.

____ Pain has restricted my social life and I do not go out as often.

____ Pain has restricted social life to my home.

____ I have no social life because of pain.

Section 10 - Traveling

____ I can travel anywhere without pain.

____ I can travel anywhere but it gives extra pain.

____ Pain is bad but I manage journeys over two hours.

____ Pain restricts me to journeys of less than one hour.

____ Pain restricts me to short necessary journeys under 30 minutes.

____ Pain prevents me from traveling except to receive treatment.

Raw score _____ **Percentage** (total score/total possible x 100) _____

Level of disability _____

Source

Reprinted from *Physiotherapy*. Vol. 66. J Fairbank, et al. The Oswestry Disability Index V2.1. Pp. 271–273. © 1983, with permission from Jeremy Fairbank, MD, FRCS.

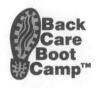

i-20

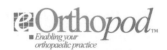

Visual Analog Scale

Name: _____   Date : _____

Place a vertical mark on the line below to indicate your present pain level.

———————————————————

      No symptoms   Severe symptoms

Source

Reprinted from *Pain*. Vol. 16. A. M. Carlsson. Assessment of Chronic Pain: Aspects of the Reliability and Validity of the Visual Analog Scale. Pp. 87–101. © 1983, with permission from The International Association for the Study of Pain.

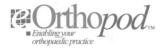

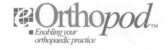

Fear-Avoidance Beliefs Questionnaire

Name: _____ Date: _____

Here are some of the things other patients have told us about their pain. For each statement, please circle the number from 0 to 6 to indicate how much physical activities such as bending, lifting, walking, or driving affect or would affect your back pain.

	Completely Disagree			Unsure		Completely Agree	
1. My pain was caused by physical activity.	0	1	2	3	4	5	6
2. Physical activity makes my pain worse.	0	1	2	3	4	5	6
3. Physical activity might harm my back.	0	1	2	3	4	5	6
4. I should not do physical activities which (might) make my pain worse.	0	1	2	3	4	5	6
5. I cannot do physical activities which (might) make my pain worse.	0	1	2	3	4	5	6

Physical activity subscale (numbers 2, 3, 4, & 5) = _____

The following statements are about how your normal work affects or would affect your back pain.

	Completely Disagree			Unsure		Completely Agree	
6. My pain was caused by my work or by an accident at work.	0	1	2	3	4	5	6

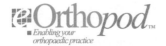

	Completely Disagree			Unsure			Completely Agree
7. My work aggravated my pain.	0	1	2	3	4	5	6
8. I have a claim for compensation for my pain.	0	1	2	3	4	5	6
9. My work is too heavy for me.	0	1	2	3	4	5	6
10. My work makes or would make my pain worse.	0	1	2	3	4	5	6
11. My work might harm my back.	0	1	2	3	4	5	6
12. I should not do my regular work with my present pain.	0	1	2	3	4	5	6
13. I cannot do my normal work with my present pain.	0	1	2	3	4	5	6
14. I cannot do my normal work until my pain is treated.	0	1	2	3	4	5	6
15. I do not think that I will be back to my normal work within 3 months.	0	1	2	3	4	5	6
16. I do not think that I will ever be able to go back to that work.	0	1	2	3	4	5	6

Work subscale = (numbers 6, 7, 9, 10, 11, 12, & 15) = _____

Total raw score (numbers 1 – 16) = _____

Source

Reprinted from *Pain*. Vol. 52. G Waddell, et al. A Fear-Avoidance Beliefs Questionnaire (FABQ) and the Role of Fear-Avoidance in Chronic Low Back Pain and Disability. Pp. 157–168. © 1993, with permission from The International Association for the Study of Pain.

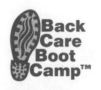

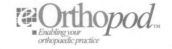

Session One: Back in Action

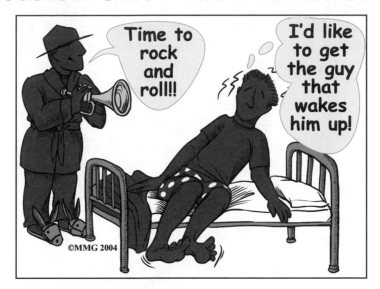

Goals for This Session

- Learn why staying active can speed your recovery.
- Learn how to take control of your condition.
- Know how to position your back to ease symptoms.
- Apply pain-relieving strategies at home.
- Begin moving safely to avoid future problems.
- Breathe properly with exercise and activity.
- Learn exercises that can help ease pain and improve mobility.

Information to Master

When back pain strikes, your first instinct may be to stop doing your normal activities for fear of pain or further injury. This session outlines the importance of gradually resuming your activity over a short period of a few days to a few weeks. You'll also get a brief introduction to spinal anatomy that will be useful as you move through the rest of the program.

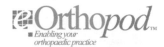

Notes

Go With the Guidelines

The best treatments for back pain are the ones that are chosen based on science. Medical scientists have compared today's research and have recommended the approaches that work the best. The final product is called a "guideline." Spine practitioners rely on these guidelines when choosing the best treatments for their patients. Guidelines for low back pain have now been developed in many parts of the world. These guidelines are similar. Here are some examples of the advice these guidelines give to patients with low back pain:

- Stay active and continue usual activities.

- Avoid bed rest for more than two days.

- Advance your activity levels over a short period of time.

- Use time, not pain, as a guide for gradually resuming activity.

- If you are working, you should stay working.

- If you are off work due to back pain, you should probably return to work sooner rather than later, using modifications when and where you need them.

Face Your Fears

Research has shown that recovery from a back problem has a lot to do with peoples' fear of pain and how they deal with it. People who have back pain may be fearful that physical or work activities will do them more harm. This fear can prevent full recovery, which helps explain why some people with back pain recover while others go on to have chronic, disabling pain.

Fear of pain is determined by a variety of factors, including personality, coping skills, and past pain and stress. Response to pain can range from confrontation to avoidance. People who face their fears (by confronting them) gradually return to their regular activities after back pain. This is seen as a healthy response. With avoidance, patients steer clear of activities they think will cause pain. This can lead to exaggerated notions of pain and increased disability over time. It can also lead to problems of inactivity, such as spine inflexibility, weakness, and weight gain.

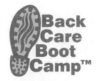
Back Care Boot Camp™

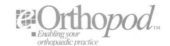
Orthopod™
Enabling your
orthopaedic practice

Avoidance behavior has been linked to more disability and work loss in people with low back pain. In fact, medical experts think that fear of pain and what we do about it may be more disabling than the pain itself. The role of "fear-avoidance beliefs" (beliefs that activities will lead to more pain and injury) can slow recovery from a back problem.

Healthcare providers can help by offering enthusiasm and instilling optimism about the positive results of treatment. They should encourage patients to get back to normal life activities by helping them overcome fear. Therapists may design a "graded" exercise program, one that helps patients gradually do a longer and harder workout. It focuses on the amount of exercise and not on the presence of symptoms. In this way patients avoid becoming inactive and are better able to get back to daily and work activities.

Take Control

There are steps you can take to keep back pain from controlling your life. Regain control of your situation by taking an active role in your recovery. Educate yourself about your condition. Learn ways to take care of back pain when it strikes. And get moving sooner, rather than later. By taking the upper hand, you'll experience a greater sense of well-being and control, leading to improved chances for early recovery.

> Successful treatment requires that you understand your condition and that you take an active role in your treatment.

Each section of your course syllabus offers ideas to help you take control of your condition. Remember you can get back to work and other normal activities swiftly. It won't cause harm and can actually help you get better faster. Learn about spine anatomy; it will help you understand why back pain happens, why a particular exercise works, and why your therapist keeps encouraging you to use proper posture and safe movement. Apply the strategies for taking care of back

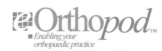

Notes

pain. And follow the advice of your therapist and doctor about staying active, even when you feel pain.

Taking control may require you to take action to improve your spine health. If you smoke, resources are available to help you quit. Because of the limited blood supply in the tissues of the low back, smoking speeds the degenerative process and impairs healing. If you are out of shape, you'll be guided in ways to get fit. Improving fitness is a key part of combating future back problems. Together, these strategies make it less likely that back pain or injury will strike again in the future.

Take Action

Passive treatments, such as rest, massage, and heat or ice, can ease pain. But they are not long-lasting if you are not also following a plan to actively resume your ordinary activities and work.

Active rehabilitation speeds recovery and reduces the possibility that back pain will become a chronic problem. Active rehabilitation involves a plan to get you back to work and play. It limits inactivity, while using active exercises (not just passive treatments). Taking action helps you resume normal activity as swiftly—and safely—as possible.

Exercising does more than help you gain flexibility, coordination, and strength. It can give you a brighter outlook in spite of your back problem. People who take part in active exercise for their back generally find it easier to do daily activities. This is because exercising actually reduces feelings of fear, disability, and depression. It gives people a sense that they really can control their pain.

Exercise therapy can help you in many ways. First, it helps you to use important muscles of the back and abdomen again. But perhaps more important, it can help you to safely do activities without hurting your back. And at its best, exercise therapy can give you the confidence to resume the tasks of your everyday life.

4

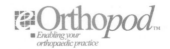

Anatomy Basics

Viewed from the side, the spine has three natural curves. The low back (lumbar spine) curves inward. The natural curves help balance and cushion the spine. A slight inward curve in the low back is called the *neutral spine position*. By learning to position your back in its neutral position, you may find that it is easier to control back pain. By resting, moving, and working with safe spine alignment, your back may feel better, and you'll be protecting your back for the years ahead.

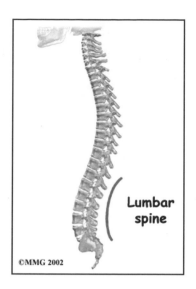

Lumbar spine

©MMG 2002

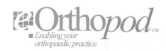

Skills to Master

Begin taking control of your back problem by mastering the following skills. These strategies are provided to supplement your visits to the clinic. Not all choices are appropriate for everyone. Perform only the items recommended by your doctor or therapist.

Positions of Comfort

Your therapist may give you ideas about how to position your back to ease pain and give the problem area a chance to heal. These positions help take pressure off the sore area by supporting your trunk or limbs.

Stomach Lying

Rationale

There is a medical myth that lying on your stomach is a bad idea when you have back pain. Certainly, it is not for everyone with back pain, but some people find that it helps to ease their back pain. Lying on your stomach can

Back Care Boot Camp™

"unload" the discs. This position can also relax muscles and improve nutrition to the structures of the back.

Description

Lie face down on a supportive mattress or couch. You may need to place a pillow under your stomach to keep your back from sagging too far forward.

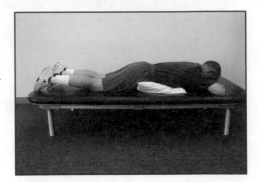

Recommendations

Follow the advice of your doctor and therapist for best results.

Concerns

If the pain in or your back or legs worsens, discontinue lying on your stomach. Be sure to notify your healthcare provider at your next clinic visit.

Back Lying

Rationale

Lying on your back with your knees supported bends (flexes) the back slightly. A flexed position of the low back takes pressure off the sore joints in the spine. It also widens the bony canals where the spinal nerve roots pass between the vertebrae, which can help take pressure off painful nerve roots. Lying on your back may also provide relief from a flare-up of low back pain.

Description

Lie on your back with your knees supported over a rolled pillow, chair, or padded box. You may be instructed to lie directly in front of a couch with your thighs pointing straight up and your lower legs resting on the seat of the couch.

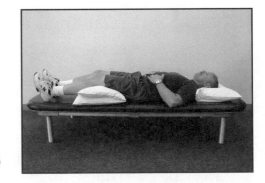

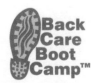
Back Care Boot Camp™

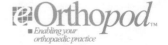
Orthopod™ ■ *Enabling your orthopaedic practice*

Recommendations

Follow the advice of your doctor and therapist for best results.

Concerns

Be aware of changes in your back or leg pain. If symptoms worsen, you may need to use a smaller bolster under your knees. If you still have pain, discontinue this position, and notify your healthcare provider at your next clinic visit.

Self-Treatments

Most patients who learn ways to take care of their back pain soon begin to self-manage their back problem. The ideas listed here are given to supplement the treatments you receive during clinic visits.

Relaxing and Breathing

Rationale

Back pain can be physically and emotionally draining. Relaxation strategies used in combination with breathing exercises can help control back pain and its accompanying stress.

Description

Deep breathing from the diaphragm helps air to reach even the lower lobes of your lungs. Deep breathing to a slow, relaxing count can help muscles relax. It also brings much-needed oxygen to sore tissues. Use one of the restful positions mentioned earlier. Turn down the lights. Put on some relaxing music. Place your hands lightly over your abdomen. Now

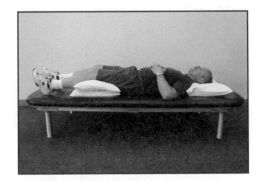

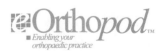

Notes

breathe slowly and deeply using your diaphragm (just under your rib cage). Feel the rhythm as your abdomen gently rises and falls. Use visual imagery to help you relax. Try to visualize each of your muscles relaxing one after another. Appropriate breathing will also be important as you begin doing other back exercises.

Recommendations

Follow the advice of your doctor and therapist for best results.

Concerns

For best results, be sure you are positioned comfortably. Avoid breathing too fast. When you complete a session of relaxing and breathing, take your time getting up. Remember that your muscles are in a relaxed state. Resume normal activities gradually.

Safe Postures

Proper sitting posture is addressed in this session. Depending on your back condition, your healthcare provider may ask you to avoid sitting whenever possible. When you do sit, support yourself with good alignment. Try not to stay in one position for too long. Take breaks often to get up, stretch out, and move around.

Sitting

Rationale

A slight inward curve of the low back balances the spine and protects it from unnecessary strain. This alignment relaxes the tissues of the spine. Awkward sitting postures, like slouching, or staying in one position for too long can make back pain worse. A balanced sitting posture can help control your symptoms and protect your back.

Description

When possible, choose a comfortable chair that supports the natural inward curve of the low back. Otherwise,

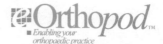

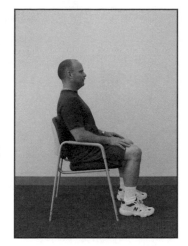

place behind your low back a rolled towel, pillow, or commercial back support. Avoid slouching by keeping your low back against the back of the chair or support. Your shoulders should be relaxed, and your hips and knees should be bent at right angles (90 degrees). Your feet should be kept flat on the floor or supported by a footrest. Avoid sitting with your legs straight out in front of you, such as when sitting in a bathtub.

Recommendations

Follow the advice of your doctor and therapist for best results.

Concerns

Sitting should be avoided when a disc is causing back problems. Studies show that sitting raises pressure markedly within the disc. Don't slouch when you sit. For example, don't sit on a soft couch where your lower spine collapses into flexion. Also, don't get stuck in one position. Get up, stretch, and move around.

Safe Movements

Taking extra care as you move during routine activities is important when controlling back pain. The strategies used to move safely are called "body mechanics."

Log Rolling

Rationale

Like a log that rolls as a single unit, the "log roll" is a way to get in or out of bed without twisting your spine. Twisting the spine, even with something as simple as getting out of bed in the morning, can put extra strain

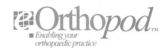

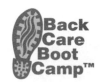

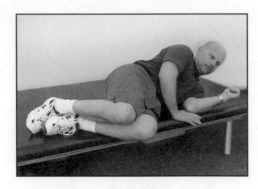

on the spine. The key to the log roll is that the spine is held steady and secure in its neutral position as you lie down and get up.

Description

To get out of bed, roll your whole body to one side as a unit, like the rolling of a log. Then let your legs ease off the edge of the bed toward the floor. At the same moment, push yourself up into a sitting position while keeping your back steady. Reverse this process when you lie down. Use this strategy during clinic visits when asked to get on or off the treatment table.

Recommendations

Follow the advice of your doctor and therapist for best results.

Concerns

When sitting up out of bed, keep your legs from dropping off the edge of the bed. You need to move slowly in order to control the movement and to keep your back in a neutral position as you sit up. If you still feel back pain when using the log roll, ask your healthcare provider to watch as you log roll. Perhaps he or she can give you additional tips to avoid pain.

Coughing and Sneezing

Rationale

Coughing and sneezing can take a toll on your sore low back. Rapid trunk flexion and forceful abdominal pressure, which are common during a violent coughing spell or sneeze, can actually herniate a weakened spinal disc. Positioning your back before you cough or sneeze may protect your back from pain and further injury.

Back Care Boot Camp™

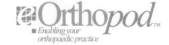

Orthopod™
■ *Enabling your orthopaedic practice*

Description

Just before you cough or sneeze, lean back slightly while placing one hand behind your back for support. At the very moment you cough or sneeze, bend your knees slightly. Another way is to place your back against a wall or door jamb as a way to keep your back straight so it doesn't lurch forward when you cough or sneeze.

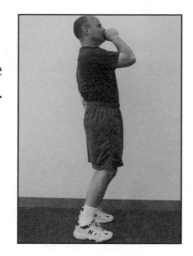

Recommendations

Follow the advice of your doctor and therapist for best results.

Concerns

A forceful cough or sneeze can cause back pain to flare. It can also put a weakened disc at risk of injury. Take a few seconds to position your back before coughing or sneezing. Let your healthcare provider know if you still feel pain or worry when you cough or sneeze.

Exercises

Exercise is vital to spine health. People who stay active after a bout of back pain do better than those who take bed rest or who limit their activity for fear of hurting their back. Even basic exercises can be used to get you moving safely. Safe exercises promote healing and control pain. Follow the advice of your therapist when doing your exercises. If pain worsens, let your therapist know during your next treatment session.

Stretches

Stretching is the basis for muscle balance in the spine. Flexibility exercises address areas of muscle tightness that may be causing a muscle imbalance. Gentle stretching is

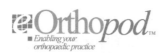

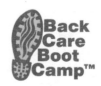

Notes

a way to relax muscles and ease pain. As your flexibility improves, you may find it easier to do other exercises and to keep better body alignment when doing your activities throughout the day.

Drill Time

Practice the skills and exercises shown by your therapist in this session. You'll be asked to demonstrate them during your next clinic visit. If you have pain or problems while practicing, your therapist can help at your next Drill Time.

Practice

Practice only the skills and exercises demonstrated by your therapist. Don't create your own exercises or go on to the next level without talking to your therapist.

Positions of Comfort

- Stomach lying
- Back lying

Posture

- Sitting

Safe Movement

- Log rolling
- Coughing and sneezing

Exercise and Stretches

- Home exercise and stretching program

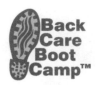

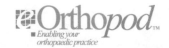

Questions for Review

1. Why is it better to try and get back to ordinary activity and employment within a short period after back pain strikes?

2. What can you do to take control of your back condition?

3. How do passive treatments and active rehabilitation differ?

Think about these questions. They will be reviewed at the start of your next session.

Session Review

Take an active role in your recovery.

- Stay active and continue usual activities.

- Avoid resting in bed for more than two days.

- Advance your activity over a short period of a few days to a few weeks.

- Use time, not pain, as your guide while you gradually resume ordinary activities.

- If you are working, you should stay working.

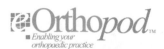

Notes

- If you are off work due to back pain, you should probably get back to work sooner rather than later, with modifications to your work if needed.

Learn all you can about your condition.

- People who educate themselves tend to have a sense of well-being and control over their situation.

- Use the syllabus as your educational guide to better back health.

Use the neutral spine position.

- Assume a slight inward curve in your low back.

- Use this position when you rest, move, lift, and work.

Begin to self-manage your back pain.

- Use safe postures to control pain and protect your back.

- Do the exercises given by your healthcare provider to help you control pain and begin moving safely.

14

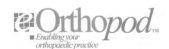

Session Two: Take Your Position

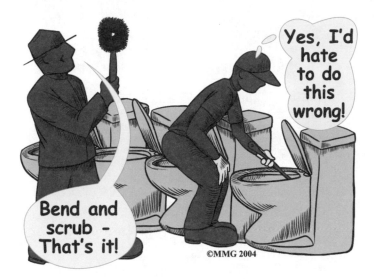

Goals for This Session

- Know the key parts of the spine.
- Apply your knowledge of anatomy to help you safely position your spine.
- Learn ways to move safely.
- Begin an aerobic exercise program.
- Master your exercises.

Information to Master

In Session One, you were shown the importance of gradually increasing your activity. The information you'll begin mastering in this session includes a detailed explanation of spine anatomy. This information will help you know how to position your spine for maximum comfort and protection. It'll also help as you position yourself for moving, lifting, and exercising.

Before jumping ahead, spend some time recalling what you learned in Session One. Review the answers to last session's Questions for Review.

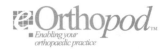
Enabling your orthopaedic practice

Back Care Boot Camp™

Notes

Answers for Review

In the last session, you were asked three questions. Take a few moments to compare your answers to those given here.

1. Why is it better to try and get back to ordinary activity and employment within a short period after back pain strikes?

People with back pain who limit their activities because they fear more pain or injury run the risk of chronic (long-term) back pain. This "avoidance behavior" has been linked to more disability and work loss in people with low back pain. By limiting activity, such as staying in bed longer than two days, muscles weaken and the body becomes unfit. People who resume activities in a short period of a few days to a few weeks tend to recover more quickly.

2. What can you do to take control of your back condition?

Take an active role in your recovery. Educate yourself about your condition. Learn ways to take care of back pain when it strikes. And get moving sooner, rather than later. You'll experience a greater sense of well-being and control, leading to improved chances for an early recovery.

3. How do passive treatments and active rehabilitation differ?

Passive treatments, like rest, massage, and heat or ice, don't require any action on your part. Used alone, passive treatments often don't have any long-term benefit. They work best when you also follow advice and a plan to actively resume your ordinary and work activities. By contrast, active rehabilitation speeds recovery because you take an active role in your therapy. It combats inactivity through exercises for key muscles, giving you confidence to be active again.

Back Care Boot Camp™

Orthopod™
■ *Enabling your orthopaedic practice*

Anatomy

The human spine is made up of 24 spinal bones, called *vertebrae*. Vertebrae are stacked on top of one another to create the *spinal column*.

As you'll recall from Session One, the spinal column has three natural curves when viewed from the side. These curves help balance and cushion the spine. The neck and low back curve inward. An inward spinal curve is called *lordosis*. The midback curves outward, called *kyphosis*.

The low back (*lumbar spine*) is made up of the lower five vertebrae. Doctors often refer to these vertebrae as L1 to L5. The lowest vertebra of the lumbar spine, L5, connects to the top of the *sacrum*, a triangular bone at the base of the spine that fits between the two pelvic bones.

Each vertebra is formed by a round block of bone, called a *vertebral body*. A bony ring attaches to the back of each vertebral body. The ring is made of the *lamina* and *pedicle* bones. When the vertebrae are stacked on top of each other, the rings form a hollow tube of bone, called the *spinal canal*. The spinal canal surrounds the spinal cord as it passes through the spine. Just as the skull protects the brain, the bones of the spinal column protect the spinal cord.

Bones of the Spine

- The spine is formed by 24 spine bones, called *vertebrae*.
- Stacked up, they form the *spinal column*.
- The spine has three natural curves.
- The lumbar spine is made up of the lowest five vertebrae and forms a slight inward curve (*lordosis*).
- A bony ring connects to the back of each vertebra, creating a hollow tube that protects the spinal cord.

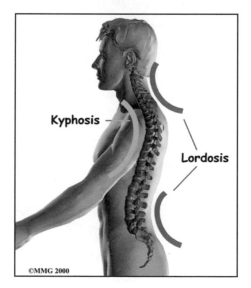

Kyphosis

Lordosis

©MMG 2000

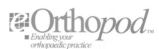

Notes

As the spinal cord travels from the brain down through the spine, it sends out nerves on the sides of each vertebra called *nerve roots*. These nerve roots join together to form the nerves that travel throughout the body and form the body's electrical system.

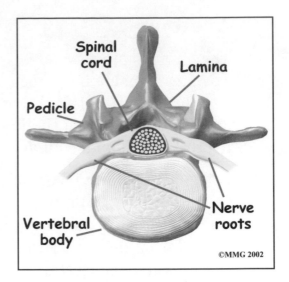

It is sometimes easier to understand what happens in the spine by looking at a *spinal segment*.

A spinal segment includes two vertebrae separated by an *intervertebral disc*, the nerves that leave the spinal cord at that level, and the small joints that link each level of the spinal column.

The intervertebral disc sits between two vertebrae. The disc is made up of two parts. The center, called the *nucleus*, is spongy. It provides most of the disc's ability to absorb shock. The nucleus is held in place by the *annulus*, a series of strong ligament rings surrounding it. *Ligaments* are strong connective tissues that attach bones to other bones.

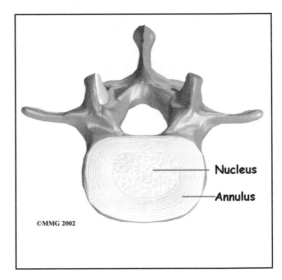

Between the vertebrae of each spinal segment are *facet joints*. The facet joints are located on the back of the spinal column. There are two facet joints between each pair of vertebrae, one on each side of the spine. The surfaces of the facet joints are covered by *articular cartilage*. Articular cartilage is a smooth, rubbery material that covers the ends of most joints. It allows the bone ends to move against each

18

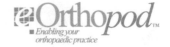

other smoothly, without friction.

The lumbar spine is supported by ligaments and muscles. The ligaments are arranged in various layers and run in multiple directions. The back muscles are also arranged in layers. Those closest to the surface are covered by a thick tissue called *fascia*. The middle layer, called the *erector spinae*, has long and thin muscles that run up and down over the ribs and low back. They come together in the lumbar spine to form a thick tendon that binds the bones of the low back, pelvis, and sacrum. The deepest layer of muscles connects along the back surface of the vertebrae. The muscles also connect the low back, pelvis, and sacrum. These deep muscles coordinate their actions with the muscles of the abdomen to help hold the spine steady during activity.

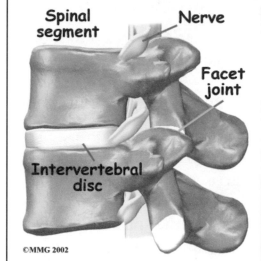

©MMG 2002

The Spinal Segment

- Two vertebrae, one on top of the other

- A disc between the two vertebrae

- Two nerves that leave the spinal cord at each level, one on the left and one on the right

- The small facet joints that link the two vertebrae together

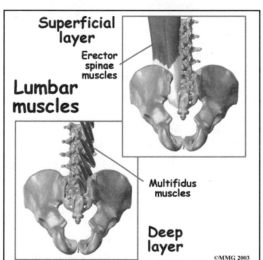

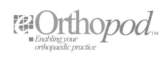

■ Enabling your orthopaedic practice

Notes

Anatomy in Action

Your knowledge of anatomy gives you a new advantage. Now you'll know how—and why—to position your spine for improved comfort. Putting anatomy into action also protects your spine from abnormal and excessive stress and strain.

Here's why. Bones, joints, and muscles work best when they are centered. If they are bent or stretched too far in one direction, they are not centered. They are out of balance. Strain from this imbalance can make your back pain worse. Centering the spine in its neutral alignment (slight lordosis) is generally a safer position and one that helps take pressure off sore areas of your back.

When the parts of the spine are out of balance, they don't work as well. For example, a muscle is weakest when it is stretched out or when it is already contracted (shortened) all the way. The same muscle is strongest between the two extremes of being stretched or shortened all the way. The muscles of the low back and abdomen work best when the spine is kept in its neutral position.

Using imbalanced spine postures upsets lifelong spine health. The strain from these imbalances may not be felt at first. But with time, they can take a toll on the parts of the spine and one day become a back problem.

To illustrate, look at your hands. Notice that the fingers are in a balanced position, curving gradually from the back of the hand to the finger tips. Now bend and hold one of your fingers gently backward. At first, the stretch you feel in your bent finger may actually feel good. However, because your finger is in an awkward alignment, one that is not "centered," you'll eventually begin to feel discomfort. Keep it there for too long, and the discomfort will give way to actual pain. The pain eases when you let go and allow the finger to resume its balanced position again.

The same is true for your back. Imbalanced spine postures may not feel like they're a problem. You might actually feel comfortable at first, such as when you sit or work with

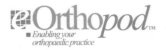

slouched posture. But with time, the small strains on the spine begin to add up. Eventually damage occurs.

The discs are affected by the position of your spine. When you bend forward, the front of the discs are squeezed as the vertebrae above and below get closer together. This pressure pushes the nucleus in the middle of the disc backward against the annulus (the ligament ring around the nucleus). If the annulus is weak, the nucleus can squeeze through, causing a disc bulge or disc herniation. The opposite pressure occurs with back bending; the nucleus pushes forward. Positioning the spine in neutral keeps the nucleus centered inside the disc.

Go Neutral

Low back posture depends on the position of your pelvis. You can change the alignment of your low back by rolling your pelvis back and forth. For example, tilting your pelvis forward pushes your buttocks out (extension). Tilting your pelvis backward pulls your buttocks in (flexion). When the lower spine is centered between the two extremes of extension and flexion, it is in neutral. Use the neutral position as you rest, move, and exercise.

Skills to Master

Continue taking control of your back problem by mastering the following skills. These strategies are provided to supplement your visits to the clinic. Not all choices are appropriate for everyone. Perform only the items recommended by your doctor or therapist.

Positions of Comfort

In Session One, you were shown rest positions to help the problem area heal. Recall that stomach lying tends to help with disc problems, whereas back lying with support takes pressure off sore facet joints and nerve roots. The positions listed in this session are beneficial because they promote the neutral spine position.

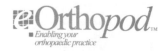

Notes

Side Lying

Rationale

Side lying may be used to position your back comfortably. It helps align your back in the middle of the spine's range of motion—between the extremes of flexion and extension. The neutral position is often ideal for reducing pressure on painful structures of the spine. And it is ideal for moving a fresh blood supply into the painful area, while moving swelling out.

Description

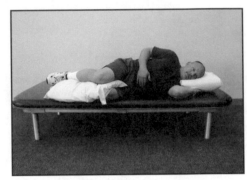

Lie on your side with your back straight and a pillow placed between your bent knees. A second pillow can be wedged behind your back to keep your trunk from rolling backward. Keep your neck in line with the rest of your spine by placing a supportive pillow under your neck.

Recommendations

Follow the advice of your doctor and therapist for best results.

Concerns

Avoid curling into a ball, which causes the low back to bend too far. Also, if you rest on a mattress or couch that is not firm, your trunk will bend as it sags into the soft surface. You may need to place a rolled towel under your side to keep your spine lined up.

Sleeping

Rationale

Getting good sleep is vital to spine health. Pain and stiffness felt when you wake up may be due to your mattress. If the mattress is too soft, your spine will sag

Back Care Boot Camp™

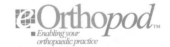
■ *Enabling your orthopaedic practice*

into the soft surface. A firm surface makes it easier to align your spine in the neutral position.

Description

Sleep on a firm mattress. If your mattress is not firm, a rolled towel wrapped around your waist can protect your back from sagging. You may find additional relief by lying on your back with your knees supported over a pillow, or by lying on your side with a pillow between your knees.

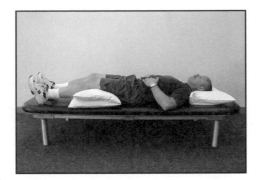

Recommendations

Follow the advice of your doctor and therapist for best results.

Concerns

Sleeping on a soft surface may partly explain unwanted back stiffness when rising in the morning. If you've tried to support your back as described above but are still awakening with back pain and stiffness, ask your doctor or therapist for other helpful tips.

Safe Postures

Proper posture is essential to spine health. When possible, keep a slight inward curve in your low back. Avoid awkward postures, such as bending or twisting the spine. Try not to stay in one position for too long. Take breaks often to get up, stretch out, and move around. The idea is to avoid too much strain on your back. In Session One, you were shown proper sitting posture. In this session, apply your understanding of spine alignment when you are standing to keep your back pain to a minimum and to give you ways of preventing future back problems.

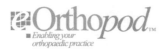

Enabling your orthopaedic practice

Back Care Boot Camp™

Standing

Rationale

A slouched standing posture is seen when the knees are kept straight, the shoulders droop or round forward, and the head and neck jut forward. Combined with the effects of gravity, this slouched posture forces the back muscles to work extra hard to keep the upper body upright. Balancing the head atop the spine and keeping a slight inward curve in the low back reduces this strain and protects against back pain and future back injury.

Description

Good standing posture doesn't mean that you stand like a soldier at attention. Rather, it is a relaxed upright position. It begins by "thinking tall." Place a hand on your chest, just below your neck. Feel your chest move from a slouched to an upright position. Find a midway point. Now roll your shoulders back slightly. Don't thrust yourself back at the waist. Instead, get into a position where you feel a slight inward curve in your low back. This standing posture balances the spine for improved efficiency and comfort. If you must stand for a prolonged period, you can keep your back relaxed by placing one foot on a step or stool. For example, when washing dishes at a sink with a lower cabinet, swing the lower cabinet door open, and place your foot on the ledge inside the cabinet.

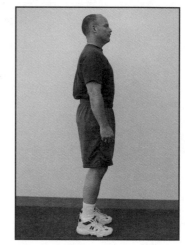

Recommendations

Follow the advice of your doctor and therapist for best results.

Back Care Boot Camp™

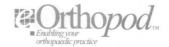
Orthopod™
■ *Enabling your orthopaedic practice*

Concerns

Wear comfortable and supportive shoes. Avoid shifting all your weight onto one foot. Instead, stand with equal weight on both feet. Also, don't get stuck in one position. Change positions; do some stretches; move around.

Safe Movements

You were introduced in session one to the "log roll" as a way to help you get in and out of bed safely. And you learned tips on how to cough or sneeze to avoid further back pain or injury. Taking extra care as you move during routine activities is important when controlling back pain. It is also key to long-term spine health. Keeping the spine safely positioned as you move helps protect the parts of the spine from awkward, painful, and repeated stresses. Use the neutral position when sitting and standing.

Sitting and Standing

Rationale

You may tend to lean too far forward when sitting down or standing up. Keep your spine in neutral to avoid flexing the spine forward.

Description

As you prepare to stand up from a chair, place your feet shoulder width apart. Keep your spine aligned in neutral. Place your nose over your toes by hinging forward at the hips. Use your buttock and thigh muscles to push yourself up. Don't twist or bend too far over at the waist, which puts added strain on the lumbar spine. Reverse this process when preparing to sit down.

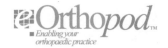

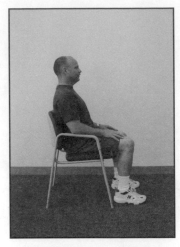
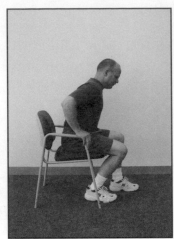
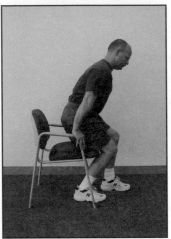
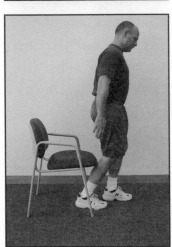

Recommendations

Follow the advice of your doctor and therapist for best results.

Concerns

Keep your back in neutral. Lean forward at the hips—not your back—when you sit or stand. If your thigh and hip muscles are weak, choose a chair with armrests so you can use your arms for additional leverage.

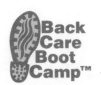

Back Care Boot Camp™

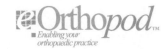
Orthopod™
Enabling your
orthopaedic practice

Notes

Self-Treatments

In Session One, you learned to control pain through proper breathing and relaxation. Applying ice or heat is another measure you can use to manage your condition, especially if symptoms are particularly bad.

Applying Ice

Rationale

Ice makes blood vessels narrow (called *vasoconstriction*). This is ideal for stopping the pain that often comes with inflammation. It can easily be used as part of a home program. Ice is especially helpful in the early hours and days after onset of back pain. Ice may also help reduce swelling, which in turn takes pressure off pain sensors within the tissues of the spine. The goal is to ease discomfort so you can rest, move, and exercise easier.

Description

Ice packs or a bag of ice are the most effective forms of cold therapy. Cold treatments usually involve applying ice to the sore area for 15 to 20 minutes. You may find you have less pain and better mobility after applying ice.

Recommendations

Follow the advice of your doctor and therapist for best results.

Concerns

Avoid injury to your skin by placing a wet towel between your skin and the cold pack or ice bag. Also, avoid heavy exercise or activity after applying cold treatments to your back. The drop in temperature can momentarily slow the responsiveness of nerves and muscles in the area, setting you up for an injury. Alert your doctor or therapist to any unusual increase in back pain.

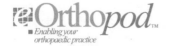

Notes

Applying Heat

Rationale

Heat makes blood vessels expand (called *vasodilation*), which helps flush away chemicals that make your back joints and muscles hurt. It also helps your back muscles relax. The goal is to ease discomfort so you can rest, move, and exercise easier.

Description

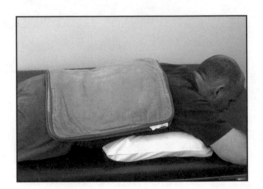

Moist hot packs, heating pads, and warm showers or baths are the most effective forms of heat therapy. Heat treatments usually involve applying heat to the sore area for 15 to 20 minutes. You may find you have less pain and better mobility after applying heat.

Recommendations

Follow the advice of your doctor and therapist for best results.

Concerns

Because heat vasodilates blood vessels, it is generally not used in the first 48 hours after the onset of back pain. Be cautious when using heat. Even when heat is the best treatment for your back discomfort, hotter is not always better. Your skin can overheat and even burn. Use layers of towels between the heat source and your skin to avoid the risk of a burn. Sleeping with an electric hot pad is a bad idea. The prolonged heat can actually burn your skin. Watch for areas of redness that don't go away within 20 minutes. This can be a sign that the temperature of the heat source is too high. Alert your doctor or therapist to any unusual increase in your back pain.

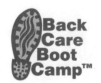

Back Care Boot Camp™

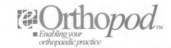
Orthopod™
■ *Enabling your orthopaedic practice*

Notes

Exercises

Continue with the exercises you received in Session One. Discuss with your healthcare provider any problems or concerns you have about your exercise program. To help you apply what you've learned about anatomy and the neutral spine, practice the two exercises outlined below.

Pelvic Tilt

Rationale

The pelvic tilt exercise helps you feel the change in low back posture that occurs with pelvic movement. It is also a gentle way to stretch the low back, while coordinating movement between the muscles of your back and abdomen.

Description

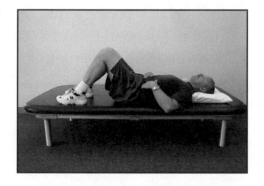

Lie on your back with your knees bent. Gently roll your pelvis back and forth. Feel how the amount of space between the mat and the small of your low back changes. As you roll your pelvis forward, you should feel the space getting larger. Your back is extending. As you roll your pelvis backward, your back flexes, making the space in the small of your back smaller. Your low back may even contact the mat as your low back flattens into flexion. Next, roll your pelvis in gradually smaller amounts until you find the middle position, between the extremes of flexion and extension. This is the neutral position. Hold this position as you close your eyes and sense what this neutral position of your spine feels like.

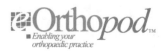

29

Recommendations

Repeat pelvic tilts 10 to 20 times slowly and gently. Practice locating and keeping the neutral position of the spine.

Concerns

Stay relaxed as you practice the pelvic tilt exercise. Keep light on your heels; otherwise your hamstring muscles on the back of your thighs will do all the work. Only roll your pelvis back and forth within a pain-free amount of movement. If you feel pain when rolling your pelvis all the way in one direction, back off slightly.

Cat and Camel

Rationale

The cat and camel exercise helps you feel the change in low back posture that occurs with pelvic movement. It is also a gentle way to stretch the low back, while coordinating movement between the muscles of your back and abdomen.

Description

Get on your hands and knees, as though you were going to crawl. Position your hips over your knees, and your shoulders over your hands. Now gently roll your pelvis back and forth. Feel how the curve in your low back changes. As you roll your pelvis backward, your back hunches into a rounded (flexed) position much like the back of a mad cat. As you roll your pelvis forward, you should feel your low back arch like that of a camel's back. Your back is extending.

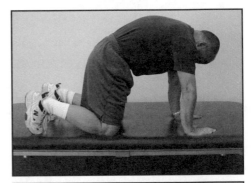

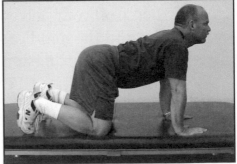

Back Care Boot Camp™

30

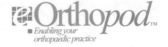

Next, roll your pelvis in gradually smaller amounts until you find the middle position, between the extremes of flexion and extension. This is the neutral position. Hold this position as you close your eyes and sense what this neutral position of your spine feels like.

Recommendations

Repeat cat and camel 10 to 20 times slowly and gently. Practice locating and keeping the neutral position of the spine.

Concerns

Stay relaxed as you practice the cat and camel exercise. Only roll your pelvis back and forth within a pain-free amount of movement. If you feel pain when rolling your pelvis all the way in one direction, back off slightly.

Stretches

Continue to do the stretches you were given in Session One. Flexibility does not happen immediately. It takes time and effort to attain muscle balance. You may find that stretching eases your pain. Discuss with your healthcare provider any problems or concerns you have about your stretching program.

Aerobic Conditioning

Current guidelines for low back pain include recommendations to begin aerobic conditioning soon after the onset of low back pain, usually within two weeks. Aerobic exercise may be recommended to help you avoid the potential debilitating effects of back pain.

There are many ways to get a good aerobic workout. Aerobic exercises include walking on a treadmill, riding a stationary bike, or swimming. These activities can relieve the stress that often goes along with low back pain, and they help your body to release *endorphins* into your blood stream. Endorphins are the body's own natural painkillers.

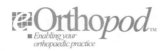

Notes

Follow your healthcare provider's advice about beginning an aerobic exercise program. At first, the goal is to gradually increase the amount of time you're doing aerobic exercise, not how hard you're working out. When you've comfortably worked up to 20 or 30 minutes during an aerobic workout, then you may be encouraged to increase the intensity of the exercise.

Drill Time

Practice the skills and exercises demonstrated by your therapist in this session. You'll be asked to demonstrate them during your next clinic visit. If you have pain or problems while practicing, your therapist can help at your next Drill Time.

Demonstrate

You may have been shown some or all of the items listed below. Go over them with your therapist to make sure you're doing them safely and correctly.

Positions of Comfort

- Stomach lying
- Back lying

Posture

- Sitting

Safe Movement

- Log rolling
- Coughing and sneezing

Practice

Use this list as a reminder of the skills and exercises you'll be practicing. Only practice the skills and exercises demonstrated by your therapist. Don't create your own

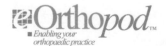

Notes

exercises or go on to the next level without talking to your therapist.

Positions of Comfort

- Stomach lying
- Back lying
- Side lying

Posture

- Sitting
- Standing

Exercise

- Pelvic tilt
- Cat and camel
- Neutral spine
- Home exercise program

Questions for Review

1. What is a spinal segment?

2. What is the neutral spine position?

3. How do the natural curves in the spine relate to the health of your back?

Think about these questions. They will be reviewed at the start of your next session.

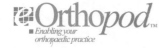

Session Review

Key points of spinal anatomy:

- Spinal bones are called vertebrae.

- The spine is formed by 24 vertebrae.

- A disc sits between each vertebral set.

- The disc has two parts: the inner nucleus, and the outer annulus.

- A bony ring on the back of each vertebra protects the spinal cord inside the spinal canal.

- Two facet joints sit between each vertebral set, one on the left and one on the right.

A spinal segment is made up of:

- Two vertebrae, one on top of the other.

- A disc between the two vertebrae.

- Two nerves that leave the spinal cord at each level, one on the left and one on the right.

- The small facet joints that link the two vertebrae together.

The spine has three natural curves.

- The neck and low back curve inward (lordosis).

- The midback curves outward (kyphosis).

- The spinal curves help balance and cushion the spine.

Spine health is maximized by keeping the spine balanced, or centered.

- When the parts of the spine are out of balance, they don't work as well.

- Using imbalanced postures upsets lifelong spine health.

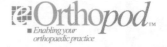

- Imbalanced spine postures may not cause pain right away.

- The neutral spine position combats abnormal and excessive strain on the back.

Aerobic exercise is an important part of recovery after back pain.

- It is recommended in most guidelines for treating low back pain.

- It can help relieve the stress that often goes along with having back pain.

- It can help keep you fit.

- It can help your body release endorphins, the body's own natural painkiller.

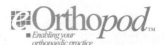

Notes

_____
_____
_____
_____
_____
_____
_____
_____
_____
_____
_____
_____
_____
_____
_____
_____
_____
_____
_____
_____
_____
_____
_____
_____
_____
_____
_____
_____
_____
_____
_____
_____
_____
_____
_____
_____
_____
_____
_____
_____
_____

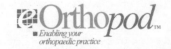

Session Three: Hold Steady

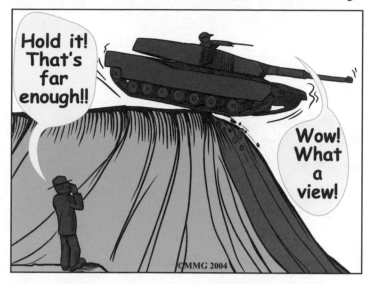

Goals for This Session

- Define *spinal stabilization*.

- Know the key stabilizers of the spine.

- Explain muscle actions that stabilize the spine.

- Begin exercises that engage key muscles of your spine.

- Learn to stabilize your spine during routine activities.

- Gradually advance the time you spend doing aerobic exercise.

Information to Master

As you learned in Session Two, the neutral position is vital to spine health. Achieving this posture while sitting or standing is one thing. It's another to know how to coordinate the muscles of your trunk and abdomen in order to support and stabilize your spine during daily and work activity. This session will give you an in-depth look at the anatomy of the spinal stabilizers. Then you'll begin to put key muscles of the back and abdomen to work during exercise and activity.

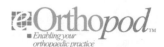

Notes

Before jumping ahead, spend time recalling what you learned in Session Two. Review the answers to last session's Questions for Review.

Answers for Review

In the last session, you were asked three questions. Take a few moments to compare your answers to those given here.

1. What is a spinal segment?

A spinal segment includes two vertebrae separated by a disc, the nerves that leave the spinal cord at that level, and the small facet joints that link each level of the spinal column.

2. What is the neutral spine position?

The neutral spine position is a comfortable back posture that is between the extremes of spine flexion and extension. In general, this middle position is a slight inward curve in the small of the back.

3. How do the natural curves of your spine relate to the health of your back?

The natural curves place the spine in a centered position, one that helps avoid extra strain on the parts of the back. The natural curves of the spine position the muscles where they work the best. Good posture and optimal muscle function protect the spine from small amounts of damage that could otherwise add up to back pain and problems.

What is Spinal Stabilization?

The body's ability to properly align, hold, and guide the spine is called *spinal stabilization*. This does not mean holding the spine rigid. Rather, spinal stabilization is the body's way of controlling and guiding the spinal joints as they move. The mobile parts of the spine are steadied so that no harmful shifting or sliding happens between each spinal segment.

The body relies on many tissues, including nerves, ligaments, and muscles, to produce spine stability. Without support

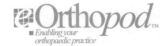

from these stabilizers, the natural curves of the spine would collapse. In this section, you'll learn the anatomy that affects spinal stability.

Why is Spine Stability Important?

As you discovered in Session Two, the spine works best and stays healthiest when it is centered in the neutral spine position. This balanced alignment reduces day-to-day strains on the parts of the spine. The strains from using poor spine postures cause small amounts of damage in the parts of the spine. You may not feel that anything is wrong. But with time, these small amounts of damage add up and may eventually cause back pain and problems.

The same thing can happen if your back isn't steady and stable as you go about daily activities. Consider the loads affecting your spine as you walk, sit, twist, lift, or carry. These actions place a demand on spinal tissues. If the spinal stabilizers are not doing their job, the loads put extra strain on the parts of the spine. This is because the spinal segment is free to shift and slide subtly. These subtle movements are not often painful. But scientists believe the wear and tear they cause can take a toll on the parts of the spine.

Anatomy of a Stable Spine

Spine stability starts with optimal alignment. Recall that the spine has three natural curves, with the low back slightly curved inward. Aligning the low back in the neutral position (between the extremes of flexion and extension) creates a stable spinal column, one that can tolerate greater loads without buckling. Spine stabilization relies on this "power position" of the low back.

You've now learned how to position your spine in neutral. The next step is to understand how the parts of your body work to keep your spine stable as you move. Safe spine

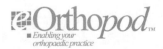

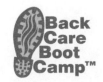

Notes

movement relies on key stabilizers of the spine. These stabilizers include

- Ligaments
- Fascia
- Muscles
- Nerves

Ligaments

Ligaments are rope-like bands of tissue that connect bones together. Most ligaments are lined up to keep joints from bending the wrong way. This feature creates stability for the joints. There are many ligaments that support and protect the joints of the low back. Several long ligaments connect on the front and back sections of the vertebrae. Smaller ligaments join one vertebra to the next. Thick ligaments also connect the bones of the low back to the sacrum (the bone below L5) and pelvis.

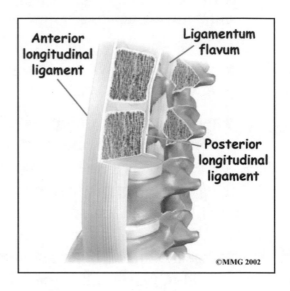

©MMG 2002

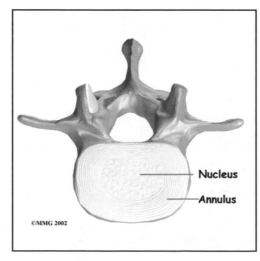

©MMG 2002

The disc (described in Session Two) also works like a big ligament. Recall that the nucleus is centered within the disc. It is surrounded by the annulus, which is a series of ligament rings. A healthy disc limits motion within the spinal segment.

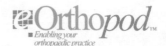

Fascia

Fascia is similar to ligaments, but fascia is more like a sheet than a rope. Fascia covers and connects muscles and organs. A large diamond-shaped sheet of fascia covers the low back. This crucial stabilizer of the lower spine is called the *thoracolumbar fascia* (TLF). Many large and important muscles connect to the TLF. As these muscles work, the TLF pulls tightly to the low back, keeping the lumbar spine from bending out of the neutral position. Because it surrounds the back muscles, the TLF also augments the power generated by these muscles.

Muscles

Spine stabilization relies on the controlled actions of many important muscles. Because of their location toward the center of the body, and because of their importance in spine stability, these key stabilizers are called "core" muscles.

Core muscles help grip and hold the spine. They keep each spinal segment from shifting and sliding as you do your activities. The two main core stabilizers are the *multifidus* and *transverse abdominal* (TA) *muscles*. Knowing where these muscles are and how they work is essential as you learn ways to stabilize your spine.

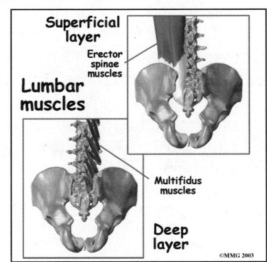

The multifidus muscles are small back muscles along each side of the spine. They come in different lengths. Some cross only from one vertebra to the vertebra below. Others cross two, three, and up to five spinal segments. In the lower spine, the multifidus muscles go from the lumbar spine to the sacrum (the bone below L5).

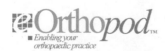

Notes

Although small, the multifidus muscles connect directly to each spinal segment, making them one of the most important muscle stabilizers of the spine.

The TA (transverse abdominal muscle) is a thin, belt-like muscle that wraps around the low back and abdomen. Think of this muscle as a girdle around your waist. As it contracts, the TA draws the lower abdomen inward, much like would happen if you were zipping up a tight pair of jeans.

Notably, this muscle anticipates your every move. The TA actually kicks in to steady the spine even before you lift an arm or leg. Scientists call this a *feed forward loop*. Nerves to the TA alert the muscle in advance of your movement, giving it a split-second advantage to grip and protect your spine. The TA's feed forward loop normally works like this. You go to grab a gallon of milk from the refrigerator. Just before you reach out your arm, your nerves signal the TA to contract. Even before you lift the milk container, your TA has already begun to engage and stabilize your spine.

Other muscles are needed for spine stability. Recall that many large and important muscles attach to the diamond-shaped sheet of fascia called the TLF. As these muscles contract, they pull the TLF tight to the back, keeping the spine in its power position. The *latissimus dorsi* muscles (the "lats") attach to each side of the top of the TLF. From there, they angle upward along your back and the sides of your upper trunk. The *gluteus maximus* muscles (the largest of the buttock muscles) connect to the lower sides of the diamond, giving the buttock and hips a solid connecting point to the TLF.

Two important abdominal muscles also connect to the TLF. One, mentioned earlier, is the TA. The other is the back portion of the *internal oblique* abdominal muscles. Training each of these key stabilizers is an important feature of your recovery—and of the future health of your spine.

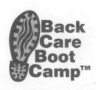

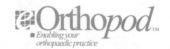

Nerves

Smooth, guided spine motion is a mark of a stable spine. Through normal nerve function, key muscles are able to keep the spine in its neutral position. These *motor nerves* signal the key muscles to grip and hold and to guide and control the spine. If the signals are not coordinated, the muscles cannot do their work to help stabilize the spine. Back pain can interrupt these signals and stop the key muscles from stabilizing the spine.

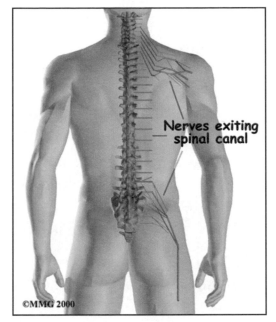

Nerves exiting spinal canal

©MMG 2000

Nerves also carry information back to the spinal cord and brain. These *sensory nerves* transmit sensations such as heat, cold, touch, pressure, and pain. They also give us our sense of position. *Position sense* tells us about our body's position. It is an essential part of the way we control our movements. Information from sensors in the skin, ligaments, tendons, muscles, and joints is sent to the brain and spinal cord about the location of our joints. We rely on position sense to locate the neutral spine position. A deficiency in our awareness of position leads to small errors in position sense and movement control, which can overload the soft tissues in the spine. When the lumbar spine can't find or keep its neutral position, movement of the spine takes place toward the extreme ends of motion rather than in the middle.

Anatomy of an Unstable Spine

How does a spine become unstable? The most obvious cause is a bad accident that tears the ligaments that support the spine. But years of poor posture and movement can also

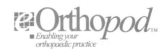
Enabling your orthopaedic practice

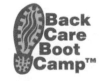

Notes

stretch spinal ligaments so that they can no longer steady the spine. An injured disc allows extra movement within the spinal segment and may create an unstable segment. Diseases that affect the supportive structures of the spine can also cause instability at one or more levels of the spine.

Altered function in the core muscles upsets spinal stability. The TA and multifidus muscles work together to grip and hold the spine, almost like an on-off switch. Back pain short-circuits this switch, and the core muscles stop working normally. The multifidus muscles that cross the problem area of the spine become sluggish and begin to shrink (atrophy). The TA shuts down, too. Its actions are no longer coordinated. When the TA and multifidus muscles are not functioning, the spine is left unprotected against daily strains.

Scientists have learned that even one instance of back pain can alter normal function in these two important core stabilizers. The problem is intensified in people with chronic back pain.

Ways to Stabilize the Spine

When the spine is unstable, there are only a few ways to make it stable again. The most dramatic way to create stability is by *lumbar fusion*, a type of back surgery that uses bone grafts and metal hardware to bind one or more spinal segments together.

A less invasive choice is a flexible back brace. Clinicians are generally not keen on issuing braces like this, however. Scientific studies have not proven that they work all that well. Such braces can help early in a course of back pain and are sometimes recommended when back pain first strikes. They are occasionally used when the back needs some added support. In these cases, they bind the back and abdomen, keeping the lower spine from extra movement. They also give patients a reminder of proper body alignment and posture.

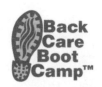

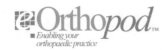

Patients who need additional lumbar stability may benefit from a flexible back brace while doing challenging activities, such as heavy lifting, hiking, and raking. However, healthcare providers will usually only issue a brace with clear instructions to remove it often to do exercises for the back and abdomen. Otherwise, these key muscles begin to rely on the brace and may begin to atrophy and weaken. Another drawback is that these braces may give a false sense of strength and security that could lead a person to over-do and possibly end up causing more damage.

A third option to support and stabilize the spine is exercise—but not just any exercise. The exercises designed to improve spine stability are often called *core stabilization exercises*. There are many variations of core stabilization exercises. In general, they usually start out easy and become more challenging as you progress. Patients who do these exercises often report improved pain control, mobility, and function.

Skills to Master

Continue taking control of your back problem by mastering the following skills. These strategies are provided to supplement your visits to the clinic. Not all choices are appropriate for everyone. Perform only the items recommended by your doctor or therapist.

Core Exercises

Your therapist may work with you to help "flip the switch" to your multifidus and transverse abdominal (TA) muscles. Getting these muscles to coordinate their efforts may seem impossible at first. Your therapist can help by using electrical stimulation over your low back to get the multifidus muscles working again. In some cases, biofeedback may be used to help you keep your back positioned and to keep you from

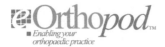

compensating with other muscles. The goal at first is to lightly contract these muscles and hold for 10 seconds or so. When you get the hang of it, you may be instructed to do several contractions often throughout the day.

Multifidus Muscle Activation

Rationale

The multifidus muscles cross each spinal segment, making them one of the best muscles to help stabilize the spine. People who've had back pain, even once, may lose the ability to work the multifidus muscles in the problem area. If the multifidus muscles aren't working right, the problem segment is left unprotected and is free to shift around during daily activities.

Description

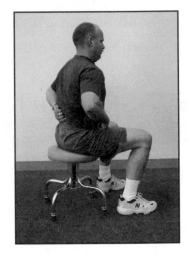

Sit with your low back in the neutral position. Reach one or both hands behind your low back. Place one or more fingers up and down the sides of your lower spine, just next to the bony bumps in the center of your low back. Gently tap or press on the multifidus muscles as shown by your therapist. Attempt to lightly engage the muscle under your fingers.

Recommendations

Hold the contraction for 10 seconds. Repeat five to 10 times.

Concerns

Don't get frustrated if at first you are unable to make the muscle work. And try not to work the muscle too hard, as this may cause you to compensate with other, less important muscles. If you have trouble with this

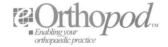

exercise, your therapist may be able to help by using other positions or treatments such as electrical stimulation or biofeedback.

TA Muscle Activation

Rationale

Recall that the TA muscles are aligned like a girdle around your waist. When they work, the TA muscles draw the abdomen in. They work with the lumbar multifidus muscles to grip and hold the spine steady. Back pain sometimes causes this muscle to either stop working altogether or to lose its ability to coordinate with the multifidus muscles. When this happens, the low back is left unprotected and at risk for further problems.

Description

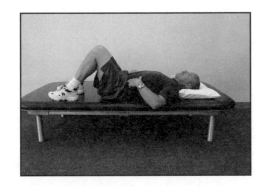

Lie on your back with your knees bent and your low back positioned in neutral. Place one hand behind your back so you can feel if your back arches or flattens during the exercise. Place your other hand lightly on your lower abdomen. The key to activating the TA muscles is to remember that they draw in the lower abdomen. As you begin to lightly contract the TA muscles, concentrate on bringing your belly button toward your spine. Breathe normally as you draw your lower abdomen in. Don't allow your abdomen to "pooch" out, as this means you are compensating with other abdominal muscles. To help activate your TA muscles, imagine you are trying to zip up a pair of tight jeans. You can improve the contraction by also working the muscles deep within your pelvis, the ones that keep you from urinating.

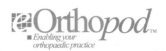

Recommendations

Attempt to lightly engage your TA muscles. Hold the contraction for 10 seconds. Repeat five to 10 times. When you get the hang of it, you may be instructed to do several contractions often throughout the day.

Concerns

Don't get frustrated if at first you are unable to make the muscle work. And try not to work the muscle too hard, as this may cause you to compensate with other, less important muscles. If you have trouble with this exercise, your therapist may be able to help by using other positions or treatments such as electrical stimulation or biofeedback.

Dynamic Stabilization

Now it's time to put your core muscles to work as you exercise and as you do your daily activities. Using your core muscles to protect your back and to guide the spinal joints during exercise and movement is called *dynamic stabilization*. Feel your muscles as they work to grip and hold your spine as you move.

Abdominal Bracing

Rationale

At first, you may simply begin working on engaging your core muscles. This action, sometimes called *abdominal bracing*, forms a starting point as you do exercises to dynamically stabilize your spine. Bracing the abdomen causes an increase in abdominal pressure, which protects and gives stability to the spine.

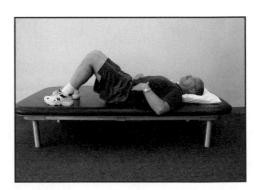

Back Care Boot Camp™

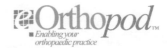
Orthopod™
■ *Enabling your orthopaedic practice*

Description

Attempt to set the muscles of your abdomen. As these muscles contract, you should feel your abdomen tighten.

Recommendations

Apply your awareness of how to engage the key stabilizers while keeping your back in its neutral position. As you gain control of the core muscles, the program advances to include more challenging arm and leg movements. Eventually, your therapist may have you do your exercises using weights, pulleys, therapy balls, foam rolls, or other methods to challenge your core and improve your spine stability. Be sure to breathe normally as you brace your abdominals.

Concerns

Don't hold your breath when you brace your abdomen, as this can cause a rise in your blood pressure. Try not to pooch out your abdomen. Instead, attempt to draw in, much like you'd feel if you were wearing a girdle around your waist.

Sit to Stand

Rationale

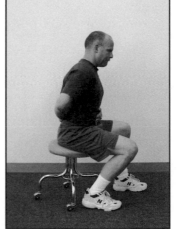

Standing up from a sitting position is a familiar activity. But have you ever stopped to think about the position of your spine as you stand up? What are your core muscles doing? Are they switched on as you move? The benefit of practicing the motion of standing from a sitting position is that you can begin to coordinate movement so that it comes from your hips, buttock, and thighs—not your low back. It also gives you a chance to work your core muscle during a dynamic activity.

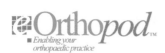
Enabling your orthopaedic practice

Back Care Boot Camp™

Notes

Description

Sit with your low back in the neutral position and your feet square on the ground, shoulder width apart. Place one arm behind your back with the back surface of your hand resting on your low back. Put your other hand lightly on your abdomen. Begin to lean forward while keeping your back in the neutral position. As you lean forward and back, you're movement should be coming from the hips and not your low back. If you feel your back rounding as you lean forward, your motion is coming from your low back, which means you're not staying in the neutral position as you move. When you've leaned forward and are in the neutral position, engage your core muscles. Now stand up. Reverse these steps when returning to a sitting position.

Recommendations

Practice this exercise several times during the day and whenever you get in and out of a sitting position. At first, you may need to watch in a side-view mirror. You'll quickly be able to see if your back position stays in neutral as you stand up and sit down.

Concerns

The tendency when standing up is to throw your weight forward, allowing your back to round. You also need to remember to "set" your core muscles to grip and hold your spine steady as you perform this familiar activity.

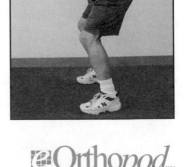

Hinged Squat

Rationale

The hinged squat exercise is a way for you to practice moving while keeping your back positioned in neutral. It's also a good way to get a workout for your hips, buttocks, and thigh muscles.

Orthopod™
■ *Enabling your*
orthopaedic practice

Description

Stand with your feet positioned just slightly wider than your shoulders. Align your back in neutral. Place one arm behind your back with the back surface of your hand resting on your low back. Put your other hand lightly on your abdomen. Next, draw your abdominals in, setting your core muscles. Now "hinge" forward by bending slightly at your hips and by bending your knees. Feel your trunk with your hands as you move to make sure your back stays in neutral.

Recommendations

Practice this exercise several times during the day and any time you need to reach for objects while bending toward the floor. At first, you may need to watch a side-view in a mirror as you do the exercise. You'll quickly be able to see if your back position stays in neutral as you move. Advance the exercise by using hand-held weights as directed by your therapist.

Concerns

The aim is to engage your core muscles, while keeping your back in neutral as you bend and reach down. Use this strategy to protect your spine as you do your routine activities.

Self-Treatments

In earlier sessions, you learned to control pain through proper breathing and relaxation and by using heat or ice. Your therapist may show you how to massage areas of your back that you can reach. Or your therapist may invite you to bring a friend or family member to get a few tips on how to give you a simple and effective back massage.

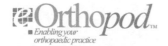

Notes

Massage

Rationale

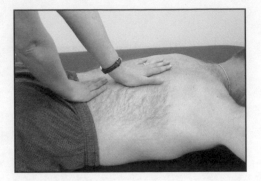

Massage can calm pain and spasm by helping muscles relax, by bringing in a fresh supply of oxygen and nutrient-rich blood, and by flushing the area of swelling and chemical irritants that come from inflammation. The idea is to help you move with less pain.

Description

Your therapist may show you or your caregiver ways to gently massage your back. Gentle strokes are best at first. These strokes can easily be done with the palms of the hands or the fingers. Use a nongreasy lotion to reduce friction during the massage. You may note the benefits of massage with a session of 10 to 30 minutes.

Recommendations

Follow the advice of your doctor and therapist for best results.

Concerns

Massaging too deeply into the sore tissues can produce soreness. If your pain increases afterward and lasts for more than an hour, the massage may have been too aggressive. Be sure to use some type of lotion to avoid friction on the skin.

Exercises

Modern guidelines for treating low back pain suggest the value of gradually progressing in an exercise program. Your therapist will help you safely advance the exercises for your core stabilizers.

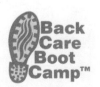

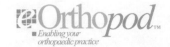

Aerobic Conditioning

Continue to carefully increase the time you are spending during your aerobic workout. Remember that it's more important at first to progress your time, not the intensity of your aerobic workout. When you've comfortably worked up to 20 or 30 minutes during an aerobic workout, then you may be encouraged to increase the intensity of the exercise.

Drill Time

Practice the skills and exercises shown by your therapist in this session. You'll be asked to demonstrate them during your next clinic visit. If you have pain or problems while practicing, your therapist can help at your next Drill Time.

Demonstrate

You may have been shown some or all of the items listed below. Go over them with your therapist to make sure you're doing them safely and correctly.

Positions of Comfort

- Stomach lying
- Back lying
- Side lying

Posture

- Sitting
- Standing

Exercise

- Pelvic tilt
- Cat and camel
- Neutral spine
- Home exercise program

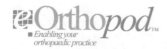

Notes

Practice

Use this list as a reminder of the skills and exercises you'll be practicing. Practice only the skills and exercises demonstrated by your therapist. Don't create your own exercises or go on to the next level without talking to your therapist.

Dynamic Stabilization

- Abdominal bracing
- Sit to stand
- Hinged squat

Exercise

- Home exercise program

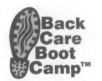

54

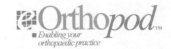

Questions for Review

1. Which four tissues in the body must work together to stabilize the spine?

2. Which two core muscles help stabilize the spine, and how do they work?

3. What are the basic principles of spinal stabilization exercises?

4. What methods are available to stabilize the spine?

Think about these questions. They will be reviewed at the start of your next session.

Session Review

What is spinal stabilization?

- It's the body's ability to properly align, hold, and guide the spine.

- It's the body's way of controlling the spinal joints as they move.

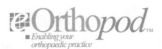
Enabling your orthopaedic practice

Back Care Boot Camp™

Notes

Why is spinal stabilization important?

- This balanced alignment reduces day-to-day strains on the parts of the spine.

- An unstable spine allows small shifts and movements in the spinal segment.

- Spinal stabilization protects against small amounts of damage that could otherwise add up to create back pain and problems.

The body relies on at least four tissues for spine stability.

- Ligaments protect the spine from unwanted movement.

- Fascia, such as the TLF in the low back, provides a connecting point for important muscles. The TLF helps keep your back in the power position and augments the power generated in your low back muscles.

- Muscles are the main dynamic stabilizers of the low back. Two key muscles are the lumbar multifidus and the transverse abdominal muscles.

- Nerves send and receive information needed to keep your spine stable. Back pain can interrupt normal nerve function, leading to impaired position sense and muscle activity.

Two core muscles work together to create spine stability.

- The transverse abdominal (TA) muscles circle the waist like a girdle.

- They coordinate their actions to grip and hold the spine.

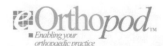

- The TA works on a "feed forward loop," giving it a split-second advantage to establish spinal stability before you actually move, lift, or do other motions.

- The multifidus muscles cross each spinal segment, making them some of the best muscles to stabilize the spine.

- The TA and multifidus muscles work together to prevent shifting between the spinal segments and to guide and control the spine as you move.

Core stabilization exercises help you recover.

- They can help by improving pain control and by giving you more mobility and function.

- They help protect the parts of the spine and lower the chance of future back pain and problems.

Flexible back braces have benefits and drawbacks.

- Benefits

  - They may help with pain control early in a course of back pain.

  - They bind the back and abdomen and help to protect against unwanted motion.

  - They can give a reminder of good alignment and posture.

  - They add some support when doing challenging activities such as raking or hiking.

- Drawbacks

  - They can cause the muscles of the back and abdomen to *atrophy* (shrink).

  - They may give a false sense of security, setting the wearer up for additional injury.

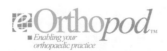

Notes

_____
_____
_____
_____
_____
_____
_____
_____
_____
_____
_____
_____
_____
_____
_____
_____
_____
_____
_____
_____
_____
_____
_____
_____
_____
_____
_____
_____
_____
_____
_____
_____
_____
_____
_____
_____
_____
_____
_____
_____
_____
_____
_____
_____

58

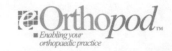

Session Four: Ready, Set, Lift!

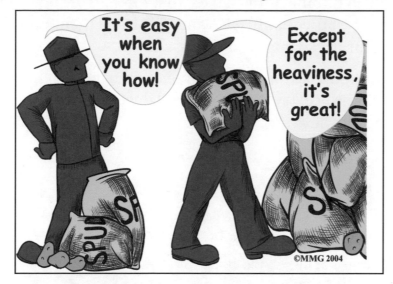

Goals for This Session

- Know how spine anatomy affects safe lifting.
- List eight "rules" to maximize back safety when lifting.
- Learn to stabilize your spine during lifting activities.
- Demonstrate safe lifting techniques.
- Perform exercises to strengthen your spine for improved lifting.

Information to Master

In Session Three, you learned how spinal stabilization can help protect your spine. You saw how the body's anatomy works to create stability, including the actions of key muscles that stabilize the spine. To lift safely, it is important that you use these muscles every time you lift.

You'll find in this session that doing a lot of lifting, lifting heavy loads, and using improper lifting technique are considered to be risk factors for back pain. However, you'll also discover that there are other factors that may have an even bigger role in how lifting influences back pain. This

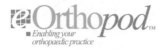

Notes

session will give you an in-depth look at how to protect your back when you lift, including a checklist for safe lifting. You'll practice using your core muscles and safe movement patterns to protect your back when you lift.

Before jumping ahead, spend time recalling what you learned in Session Three. Review the answers to last session's Questions for Review.

Answers for Review

In the last session, you were asked four questions. Take a few moments to compare your answers to those given here.

1. Which four tissues in the body must work together to stabilize the spine?

Ligaments protect the spine from unwanted movement. *Fascia*, such as the TLF (thoracolumbar fascia) in the low back, provides a connecting point for important muscles. It also keeps your back in the power position and amplifies the power that is generated in your low back muscles. *Muscles* are the dynamic stabilizers of the low back. *Nerves* send and receive information needed to keep your spine stable. Back pain can interrupt normal nerve function, leading to impaired position sense and muscle activity.

2. Which two core muscles help stabilize the spine, and how do they work?

Lumbar multifidus: The multifidus muscles cross each spinal segment, making them one of the best muscles to stabilize the spine. They work together with the transverse abdominal muscles to prevent shifting between the spinal segments and to guide and control the spine as you move.

Transverse abdominal (TA): The TA works on a feed-forward loop, giving it a split-second advantage to establish spine stability before you actually move, lift, or do other motions. The TA coordinates its actions with the multifidus muscles to grip and hold the spine.

3. What are the basic principles of spinal stabilization exercises?

These exercises start out by engaging the core muscles. Bracing the abdomen causes an increase in abdominal pressure, which gives added stability to the spine. Eventually, the exercises

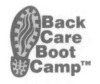

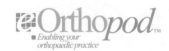

progress to include weights, pulleys, therapy balls, foam rolls, or other methods to challenge your core and improve your spine stability.

4. What methods are available to stabilize the spine?

The most dramatic way to stabilize the spine is lumbar fusion surgery, which often involves bone grafts and metal plates and screws. A less invasive measure is a flexible back brace, though there are some drawbacks that keep most spine practitioners from issuing them routinely. Finally, lumbar stabilization exercises are often prescribed as a way to train the core muscles to hold and protect the spine during activity.

Anatomy of a Safe Lift

Your knowledge of spine anatomy gives you an advantage that can help you lift safely. Recall from Session Three that spine stability starts with optimal posture, the power position. You also learned that the power position is secured by muscles that act on the thoracolumbar fascia (TLF). And you discovered that two key muscle stabilizers, the transverse abdominal and multifidus muscles, coordinate their actions to grip and hold and to guide and control the spine.

You need to keep your low back in the power position when you lift. Setting your core muscles before and during the lift tightens the TLF to your low back. This secures your back in the power position. It allows the TLF to augment the power generated by your back muscles.

Keeping your low back in its power position also requires that you bend your hips and knees when lifting. Bending forward from your hips is different than flexing your low back forward. Flexing your back causes the low back to round forward and to come out of the power position. But if you bend at the hips, you'll find that you can keep your back positioned with a slight inward curve as you bend to lift. To do this you need to hinge forward at the hips, instead of flexing your back forward. This is very similar to the exercise you learned in the last section called the "hinged squat."

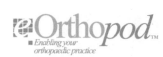

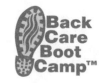

Notes

Done properly, the low back stays in the power position when you bend your hips and knees and as you hinge forward from your hips—not your low back.

Stability during lifting is improved by keeping your feet apart. This posture lowers your center of gravity and gives you a wide base of support. You rarely see a football player tip-toeing on the field. If you do, the player won't be upright very long. An opponent merely has to make contact and the player will be easily knocked down. Instead, players stay low by bending their hips and knees. In this way they are stable and can take a block or hit without getting knocked down. Likewise, your safety improves by keeping your feet apart, bending your knees, and by hinging forward with your hips.

You can give your back another advantage by keeping the load you are lifting close to your body. The further away you hold the item, the greater the forces that are multiplied to your back. Holding a 10-pound box two feet in front of you creates hundreds of pounds of force on your low back. The same box held close to your body produces less than 100 pounds of force.

Finally, avoid twisting your back when you lift, especially if you must bend to lift the object. Twisting and bending at the same time is hazardous to the parts of the back. It places extra strain on the supportive ligaments, and it increases pressure and strain on the discs of the low back.

Checklist for Safe Lifting

Follow the rules in this safety checklist to improve your safety when you lift.

Plan and Prepare

It only takes a moment to make sure your lift will be performed safely. Check to make sure you have a clear path. Remove obstacles, and avoid slippery surfaces. Before you lift, think through the steps you'll take to lift safely.

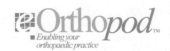

Use a Wide Base of Support

Place your feet a minimum of shoulder width apart. This position lowers your center of gravity and helps improve your stability.

Keep the Load Close

Keeping the load close to your body reduces strain on your low back. Holding the load away from your body magnifies the strain on the parts of your low back.

Use the Neutral Spine Position

Align your back in the power position, with the small of the back in a slight inward curve. Your therapist can help you find and feel what the ideal position is for the safety of your low back.

Engage Your Core Muscles

Before lifting, engage the key stabilizers of the low back and abdomen. As these muscles tighten, they'll act as a brace to hold your spine from shifting as you lift. Feel the muscles draw inward as they hold the spine steady and as they guide your spine movements while you lift.

Lift With Your Legs

To lift with your legs, keep your lower back in the power position. Bending at the hips and knees (and not your back) allows you to use the large hip and leg muscles when you lift.

Avoid Twisting

To avoid twisting as you lift, pivot your feet while moving the load from one point to the next. In other words, keep your behind where it belongs—behind you!

Get Help if Needed

If the load is too bulky or too heavy, get help from a friend or co-worker. When needed and available, use a lifting device.

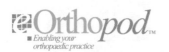

Notes

Don't get too busy and think you can't wait for help. And don't think you're tough enough to handle an unsafe situation. A strong will does not take the place of a reasonably safe lift.

Do Lifting Belts Help?

Can you lift with greater safety by wearing a lifting support belt? The answer, according to today's leading scientists, is probably not. There simply is no consistent research to show that wearing a lifting belt makes lifting any safer.

Back injuries are most effectively reduced when a complete work safety program is used. Work safety programs improve how the workplace is designed and how work is done. They also include training on how to identify unsafe lifting situations and how to use safe lifting techniques. Simply relying on a lifting support belt is not adequate protection against back injuries in the workplace.

Some doctors may prescribe a lifting support for patients who've had an episode of back pain or injury and who are returning to jobs that involve heavy and repeated lifting. In these cases, the support belt is usually issued in combination with exercises for the back and abdominal muscles, because relying on a lifting belt can cause the trunk muscles to weaken.

There are several drawbacks to using lifting support belts. First, they can create a false sense of security, giving the feeling that more can be lifted than the body can do safely. Second, there is no proof that lifting belts remind workers to keep the back lined up for safe lifting. Third, long-term reliance on lifting supports can lead to inactivity, atrophy, and weakness in the back and abdominal muscles. Fourth, an

Check the List

Plan and prepare.

Use a wide base of support.

Keep the load close.

Use the neutral spine position.

Engage your core muscles.

Lift with your legs.

Avoid twisting.

Get help if needed.

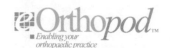

ill-fitting brace often causes the wearer to loosen the straps or laces, leading to a greater chance of back injury. Finally, lifting belts can produce a sense of psychological dependence in which the person feels he or she can't lift or work safely without wearing a lifting belt.

If your doctor or therapist recommends that you use a lifting support belt:

- Wear it properly.

- Be sure to keep all straps and laces secured.

- Avoid back injuries by making it a habit to use safe lifting techniques whether or not you are wearing a lifting support.

Risks of Lifting and Back Pain

By itself, lifting is not necessarily a risk factor for back pain. It becomes a risk for back pain when other variables are added. For example, lifting with poor technique is a risk, such as lifting when the back is bent and especially when it is twisted.

Lifting a load of unexpected or unknown weight also adds risk to the equation. The lifter may think that the item weighs more or less than it does. Getting the body ready to lift an object depends on knowing how much the item weighs. Using more force than is needed to move materials can increase the risk of falling backwards or of straining the back. The same risk applies to unstable loads or loads that shift suddenly, such as liquids.

Lifting becomes a risk for the person who has to lift over and over during the day. Lifting items for more than half of the work day poses an added risk for back pain. The risk from repetitive lifting also goes up when loads of 50 pounds or more are involved.

For some people who have had a back injury while lifting, their advice for safe lifting is to not lift at all. Yet back pain

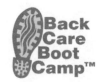

Notes

from lifting is probably somewhat overrated. Scientists do not agree that lifting (all by itself) causes back pain. More likely, lifting may only trigger the problem, making it a target of blame. There is conflicting evidence on whether people in heavy jobs actually report more back pain than people in less physical jobs.

Scientists do agree that other factors are usually involved in the onset of back pain. For example, there is some evidence that people who are overweight or who smoke may have more back pain related to lifting. And there are mental issues that affect peoples' chances of back injury at work. People who worry they'll get injured while lifting at work are at greater risk for back pain or injury. In this instance, the risk goes well beyond the task of lifting. It's the worry that raises the potential dangers of lifting.

Lifting is not always the culprit when it comes to back pain and back injury. The connection between lifting and back pain has something to do with general health, such as maintaining ideal body weight and avoiding tobacco. It also has to do with attitudes about job satisfaction, work stress, and worry about how lifting at work might hurt your back. That's why a healthy work culture reduces time lost from work due to back pain and back injuries. People can improve their back safety by improving the strength in their core muscles and by using these muscles while they lift. Using common sense helps, too.

Skills to Master

Continue taking control of your back problem by mastering the following skills. These strategies are provided to supplement your visits to the clinic. Not all choices are appropriate for everyone. Perform only the items recommended by your doctor or therapist.

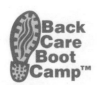
Back Care Boot Camp™

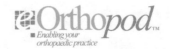
■ *Enabling your orthopaedic practice*

Safe Lifting

The "perfect lift" is one where you lower your body down by bending your hips and knees. Your back stays erect, and you hold and lift the item from directly below you. There's less force on your back, and your hips and legs do all the work—not your back muscles. But most often, you have to bend forward to get the item. This requires timing and coordination between your back and hips as you bend forward to gather and lift the item. Imagine how you would safely lift a bag of groceries from the back seat or trunk of a car, pick a bulky object off the floor, or grab a trash container from a kitchen cupboard or pantry. The skills listed here are designed to help you gain strength and coordination in your back, hips, and buttock muscles so you can keep your back safe when you lift.

Ball Squat

Rationale

The ball squat exercise coordinates timing between your back and hips. It's a way to practice lifting with your back in the power position as you bend forward with the hips and knees.

Description

Position a large therapy ball behind your back so the ball is between your back and the wall. You should be about two feet from the wall. With your back against the ball and your feet shoulder width apart, squat down by bending your hips and knees. You need to bend forward at your hips, keeping your back in contact with the ball. Allow your hips to drop back so that you hinge forward at your hips. Your arms should point straight down toward the ground, as

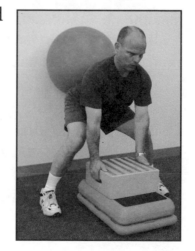

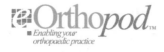
Enabling your orthopaedic practice

Back Care Boot Camp™

Notes

though you were about to grab and lift an item from the floor.

Recommendations

Keep your back in the power position. Repeat the ball squat 10 times, for two to three sets. Concentrate on timing, not speed of the exercise.

Concerns

You may have a tendency to simply squat by keeping your back straight up and down. That's not the idea. Most lifts require you to bend forward to make the lift. The ball squat is designed to get you to bend forward at the hips, while keeping your back in the power position. The action really comes from your hips. Avoid the tendency to round your back forward. Instead, keep your back in the power position at all times.

Mock Lift

Rationale

The mock lift is a way to practice lifting light objects with proper technique.

Description

Place a light object, such as a pillow or empty box, on the floor. Use the coordinated actions you practiced in the ball squat exercise to reach down and lift the object from the floor. Keep your back in the power position. Bend forward at the hips. Lower your arms toward the object by bending your hips and knees. "Set" your abdominals as you get ready to lift the item up. Return the item to the floor, and repeat the mock lift.

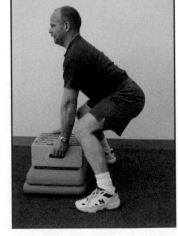

Recommendations

Imagine that the item you're lifting is quite heavy. Use safe lifting technique

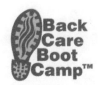

Back Care Boot Camp™

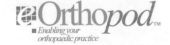

Orthopod™
■ Enabling your
orthopaedic practice

at all times. Practice five to 10 times. You may need to watch in a side-view mirror to ensure that you are hinging forward and that you are keeping your back in the power position.

Concerns

Don't just squat down with your back straight up and down. The idea is to practice hinging forward at the hips, bringing your upper body forward. This requires that your hips drop back and that you lower yourself from the hips and knees.

Lifting Styles

We are constantly faced with the need to lift items. There are a variety of lifting styles that may prove useful at different times. Practice and use the choices listed here. Your therapist may determine that one style works best for you in most situations.

Golfer's Lift

Rationale

The golfer's lift is a way to safely reach down to pick up small objects off the floor or to reach over a barrier, such as a low fence. Another option is to squat down. But let's face it. It feels sort of ridiculous to squat to the ground for something as small and light as, say, a pencil. So the golfer's lift is a nice alternative to squatting down, and it's much safer than simply bending over at the waist with your legs straight.

Description

Surely you've seen a golfer reaching into the cup after a game-winning putt. One foot stays fixed on the

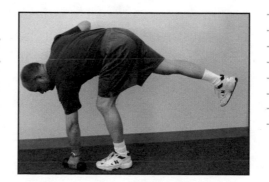

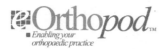
Enabling your orthopaedic practice

Back Care Boot Camp™

ground as the golfer leans forward horizontally to get the ball. The back leg points straight back to counterbalance the weight of the upper body. The back stays straight the entire time.

Recommendations

Practice the golfer's lift to pick up small items off the floor.

Concerns

To lift a light object from the floor, you may be tempted to simply keep your legs straight and bend over from your waist. Don't be fooled. This position places huge forces on your back, even if the item you're picking up is nearly weightless. The golfer's lift allows you to reach down while protecting your back. However, it requires a good bit of balance. Avoid losing your balance by holding onto the edge of a table or chair or by placing your hand firmly on your thigh.

Diagonal lift

Rationale

The diagonal lift is useful for heavier items that are close to the ground, such as a heavy box. Because this lift requires that you get down close to the item, you protect your back by making your legs do the lift.

Description

Instead of approaching an item straight on, come at it diagonally from one corner. Lower your body down and place one knee on the ground. Gather the item onto your thigh and into your lap. With your back straight and your arms secured around the item, set your core muscles, and stand straight up—making sure your head rises before your hips.

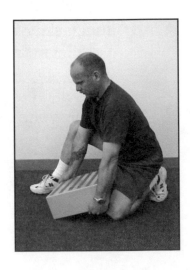

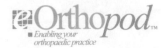

Recommendations

Practice the diagonal lift to pick up heavy items from the floor.

Concerns

You need strong legs to lift heavy items using the diagonal lift. If the item is too heavy or your legs are too weak, you may easily lose your balance during the lift. When you approach the item, first lift up one corner to see how heavy it is. If it is too heavy, get the help of a partner or a lifting device.

Power Lift

Rationale

The power lift can be used when heavier items are conveniently positioned. It protects the back by relying on the powerful and strong muscles of the hips and thighs.

Description

The power lift is similar in style to the technique used by power lifters. Position your body over the item to be lifted. Lower your body toward the item by bending your hips and knees only, keeping your back erect. Do not hunch your back forward. Grasp the item. Set your core muscles. Lift straight up by leading first with your head and then with your hips. Pull the item in close to your waist as your lift.

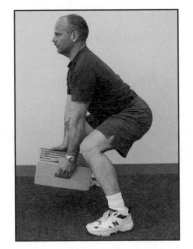

Recommendations

Practice the power lift to pick up heavy items that are conveniently located.

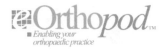
Enabling your orthopaedic practice

Notes

Concerns

Your hips, buttocks, and thigh muscles do the work during the power lift. Avoid the temptation to lift items that are heavier than you can handle. Again, get help if needed.

Lifting Strategies

The concepts you've learned in this session can be applied to a variety of lifting situations. The following examples are but a sampling of challenging areas that need attention when you lift. The key is to familiarize yourself with the concepts of safe lifting including lifting with your legs, keeping your back in the power position, and avoiding twisting. Once you've got the concepts, you can apply them to every lifting situation you encounter. Practice and use the choices listed here. Your therapist can work with you to refine strategies for these and other lifting situations.

Lifting Infants and Kids

Rationale

Unlike lifting a compact box with handles on it, children come in all shapes and sizes. They pose a unique challenge for safe lifting. They may be lying down, sitting up, flailing their arms, or waiting in a crib. The key to safely lifting infants and children is to always apply the concepts of safe lifting.

Description

Plan ahead. When possible, don't be in a hurry. Keep your back in the power position as you bend down toward the child, hinging at your hips and not hunching your back. Gather the child close to your chest. Rise up using your hip, buttock, and leg muscles.

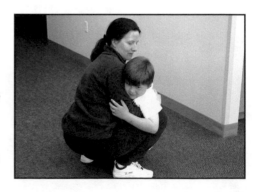

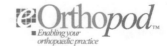

Recommendations

Remember the rules of lifting and apply them in each situation where you are lifting a child or infant.

Concerns

Your natural instincts when a child needs you may be to move quickly and not to consider the health of your back. Pause for just a moment in each lifting encounter to make sure you are safe and ready before proceeding to lift a child or infant.

Loading and Unloading a Clothes Dryer

Rationale

Getting clothes in and out of a dryer poses challenges to safe lifting. Wet clothes are heavy. And a large load requires repeated motions to get items in and out of the dryer. Using the concepts of safe lifting can help protect your spine when loading and unloading a clothes dryer.

Description

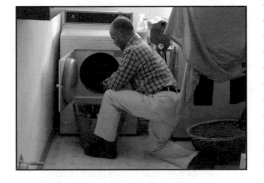

Place washed items into a clothes basket. Use good technique as you place the basket on the floor next to the dryer. To avoid twisting your back, bend down so that you are facing the front of the dryer. Kneeling on one knee is easiest. Hinge your hips forward to keep your back in the power position when placing items from the basket into the dryer. Reverse this order when removing items from the dryer.

Recommendations

Practice hinging forward and back while in a half-kneeling position. Use good technique when loading and unloading the clothes dryer.

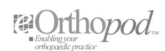
Enabling your orthopaedic practice

Back Care Boot Camp™

Notes

Concerns

It may seem easiest to simply lean sideways to load or unload the dryer. Take the needed time to position your back and to move and lift safely. Your efforts help protect your spine during routine and repeated activities.

Exercises

Today's guidelines for treating low back pain suggest the value of gradually progressing in an exercise program. Your therapist will help you safely advance the exercises for your core stabilizers. Coordinating and toning the core stabilizers is vital for improving safety when you lift.

Drill Time

Practice the skills and exercises shown by your therapist in this session. You'll be asked to demonstrate them during your next clinic visit. If you have pain or problems while practicing, your therapist can help at your next Drill Time.

Demonstrate

You may have been shown some or all of the items listed below. Go over them with your therapist to make sure you're doing them safely and correctly.

Dynamic Stabilization

- Abdominal bracing
- Sit to stand
- Hinged squat

Practice

Use this list as a reminder of the skills and exercises you'll be practicing. Practice only the skills and exercises demonstrated by your therapist. Don't create your own exercises or go on to the next level without talking to your therapist.

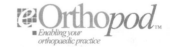

Notes

Safe Lifting

- Ball squat
- Mock lift

Lifting Styles

- Golfer's lift
- Diagonal lift
- Power lift

Lifting Strategies

- Lifting infants and kids
- Loading and unloading a clothes dryer

Exercise

- Core stabilization exercises
- Home exercise program

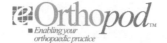

Notes

Questions for Review

1. When does lifting become a risk factor for back pain?

2. How can you protect your back when loading or unloading a clothes dryer?

3. How might you reply to a co-worker or supervisor who tells you that your back problem will be solved if you'd just wear a back brace when you lift at work?

Think about these questions. They will be reviewed at the start of your next session.

Session Review

The anatomy of your low back contributes to spine stability when you lift.

- Spine stability is maximized by using the neutral, power position of the back.

- The TLF (thoracolumbar fascia) helps keep the back in neutral and augments the power generated by the back muscles

- The multifidus and TA (transverse abdominal) muscles coordinate their actions to grip and hold and to guide and control the spine as you lift.

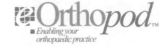

- Bending at the hips and knees helps keep your spine in the power position for lifting.

Give your back an added advantage whenever you lift.

- Lower your center of gravity by keeping your feet apart.

- Keep the load you are lifting close to your body.

- Avoid positions where your back is twisted or bent as you lift.

Keep the eight rules of lifting in mind whenever you must lift.

- Plan and prepare.

- Use a wide base of support.

- Keep the load close.

- Use the neutral spine position.

- Engage your core muscles.

- Lift with your legs.

- Avoid twisting.

- Get help if needed.

Lifting belts are not supported by modern research.

- Scientists still haven't proven that lifting support belts reduce the chances of injury.

- Lifting belts should not be relied upon to protect against back injuries in the workplace.

- They may be of some help for patients who've had an episode of back pain or injury and who are returning to jobs that involve heavy and repeated lifting.

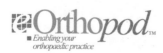

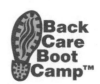

Notes

- Reliance on a lifting support belt can cause the trunk muscles to weaken.

Lifting support belts have several drawbacks.

- They can create a false sense of security.
- They haven't been proven to remind workers how to keep their backs lined up for lifting.
- They can cause atrophy and weakness in the back and abdominal muscles.
- Worn improperly, they heighten the risk for back injury.
- People can become psychologically dependent on them.

Lifting becomes a risk factor for back pain only in certain conditions.

- When the lifter uses poor technique.
- When loads of unexpected or unknown weights are lifted.
- When lifting has to be repeated, especially with loads over 50 pounds.

Other factors also make lifting a risk for back pain.

- Abusing tobacco.
- Being overweight.
- Feeling stress about work.
- Feeling dissatisfied with your job.
- Worrying that you'll get hurt lifting at work.

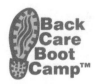

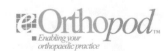

Session Five: Back Pain Basics

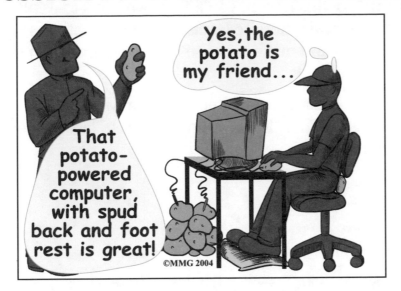

That potato-powered computer, with spud back and foot rest is great!

Yes, the potato is my friend...

©MMG 2004

Goals for This Session

- Learn the basics of the degenerative model of back pain.
- Explain the natural effects of time on the parts of the spine.
- Know the difference between mechanical and neurogenic back pain.
- Learn strategies to move and lift safely.
- Calculate workout levels during aerobic exercise.

Information to Master

In this session, you'll need to rely on your knowledge of anatomy. It will help you begin to understand the series of natural changes that occur in the spine with the passage of time. You'll start to see why back pain is common and perhaps why it has affected you. The pain that occurs from these changes is usually mechanical pain. In this session, you'll learn the difference between mechanical pain and a more concerning type of pain called *neurogenic pain*.

By now, you should be gradually advancing the amount of time you're doing aerobic exercise. Now it's time to begin

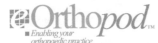

ramping up how hard you're exercising. In the Skills to Master section of this lesson, you'll find two ways to easily monitor your aerobic exercise levels. Use these methods to set realistic goals and make exercise more meaningful and fun.

Before jumping ahead, spend time recalling what you learned in Session Four. Review the answers to last session's Questions for Review.

Answers for Review

In the last session, you were asked three questions. Take a few moments to compare your answers to those given here.

1. When does lifting become a risk factor for back pain?

Recall that, by itself, lifting is not a known risk factor for back pain. Other factors that make it risky include: lifting with poor technique (bending or twisting); handling unexpected, unknown, or unstable loads; lifting for more than half the work day; lifting more than 50 pounds repeatedly; worrying about getting injured while lifting at work; being overweight; having a tobacco habit.

2. How can you protect your back when loading or unloading a clothes dryer?

Don't underestimate the amount of strain this activity can place on the low back. Remember and apply the concepts of safe lifting. Plan ahead. Position yourself by kneeling on one knee in front of the dryer. Hinge from the hips to keep your spine in the power position.

3. How might you reply to a co-worker or supervisor who tells you that your back problem will be solved if you'd just wear a back brace when you lift at work?

Today's research hasn't shown that wearing a lifting belt makes lifting any safer. By itself, a lifting belt is not helpful, but it may have some value when used in combination with a complete work safety program. Lifting belts have drawbacks. They can create a false sense of security, weaken trunk muscles, and cause psychological dependence.

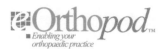

A Model for Back Pain

During an office visit for low back pain, your doctor or physical therapist may describe how changes in the spine can sometimes cause back pain. The terms *degeneration* or *degenerative disc disease* may be used. Although the parts of the spine do change with time and in some sense degenerate, this does not mean your spine is deteriorating and that you are headed for future pain and problems. These terms are simply a starting point for describing what occurs in the spine over time and how the changes may explain the symptoms you may be feeling.

Spine degeneration tends to follow a predictable pattern, or model. This pattern of changes is called the *degenerative model of back pain*. The model describes a sort of chain reaction of changes in the spine that can lead to back pain.

Recall from Session Two that the discs between the vertebrae have two parts. The inner, spongy part is the *nucleus*. The ligament that surrounds the nucleus is called the *annulus*.

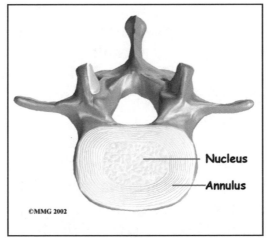

Nucleus
Annulus
©MMG 2002

The first stages of the degenerative process affect these two structures. At first, the annulus around the nucleus weakens and begins to develop small cracks and tears. The body tries to heal the cracks with scar tissue. But scar tissue is not as strong as the tissue it replaces.

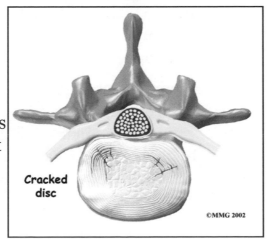

Cracked disc
©MMG 2002

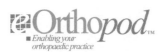

The torn annulus can be a source of pain for two reasons. First, there are pain sensors in the outer rim of the annulus. They create a painful response when the tear reaches the outer edge of the annulus. Second, like injuries to other tissues in the body, a tear in the annulus can cause pain due to inflammation.

The disc continues to change over time. At first, the disc is spongy and firm. The nucleus in the center normally contains a great deal of water, which gives the disc its ability to absorb shock and protect the spine from heavy and repeated forces. But with time, the nucleus begins to lose its water content and becomes dehydrated. The nucleus becomes thick and fibrous, so that it looks much the same as the annulus. As a result, the nucleus isn't able to absorb shock as well. Routine stress and strain begin to take a toll on the structures of the spine.

The disc loses water, causing it to lose some of its fullness and height. As a result, the vertebrae begin to move closer together, and the space between the vertebrae shrinks. This compresses the facet joints along the back of the spinal column. As these joints are forced together, extra pressure builds on the articular cartilage on the surface of the facet joints. This extra pressure can damage the facet joints. Over time, arthritis in the facet joints can develop.

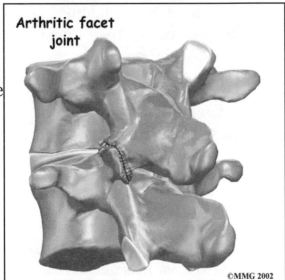

Arthritic facet joint

©MMG 2002

These degenerative changes in the disc, facet joints, and ligaments cause the spinal segment to become loose and unstable. The extra movement causes even more wear and tear on the spine. As a result, more and larger tears occur in the annulus.

Back Care Boot Camp™

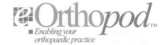
Orthopod™
■ *Enabling your orthopaedic practice*

The nucleus may push through the torn annulus and into the spinal canal. This is called a *herniated* or *ruptured disc*. The disc material that squeezes out can press against the spinal nerves. The disc also emits enzymes and chemicals that produce inflammation. Pain is caused by the combination of pressure on the nerves and inflammation caused by the chemicals released from the disc.

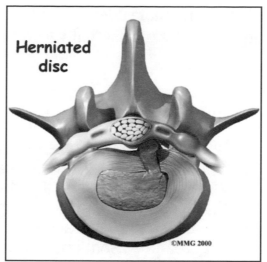

Herniated disc

©MMG 2000

As the degeneration continues, *bone spurs* develop around the facet joints and the disc. No one knows exactly why these bone spurs develop. Most doctors think that bone spurs are the body's attempt to stop the extra motion between the spinal segments.

Bone spurs can cause problems by pressing on the nerves of the spine where they pass through the openings between the vertebrae (the *neural foramina*). Pressure around the irritated nerve roots, called *foraminal stenosis*, can cause pain, numbness, and weakness in the low back, buttocks, and lower limbs and feet.

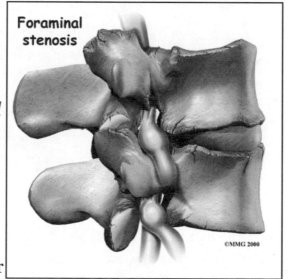

Foraminal stenosis

©MMG 2000

A collapsed spinal segment eventually becomes stiff and immobile. Thickened ligaments and facet joints, scarred and dried disc tissue, and protruding bone spurs prevent normal movement. Typically, a stiff joint doesn't cause as much

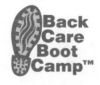

Back Care Boot Camp™

Orthopod™
Enabling your orthopaedic practice

Notes

pain as one that slides around too much. So this stage of degeneration may actually lead to pain relief for some people.

Natural History of Low Back Pain

Most back problems come from wear and tear on the parts of the spine over many years. This process is called *degeneration*. Over time, the normal process of aging can result in degenerative changes in all parts of the spine. These are natural changes that happen with the passing of time. Some people experience pain from these changes; others don't. Here's a brief overview of spine changes that tend to occur over time:

• At first, the annulus weakens, tears, and scars.

• The nucleus begins to lose water content.

• As disc height decreases, the vertebrae move closer together.

• This puts pressure on the facet joints, which can cause these joints to become arthritic.

• Changes in the ligaments, discs, and facet joints can cause the spinal segment to become loose and unstable.

• The nucleus may squeeze (herniate) through the weakened annulus.

• Bone spurs form on the vertebrae.

The spine changes described here occur with age, much like our hair turns gray. Conditions such as a major back injury or fracture can affect how the spine works, making the changes happen even faster. Daily wear and tear and certain types of vibration can also speed up degeneration in the spine. In addition, strong evidence suggests that smoking

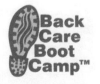

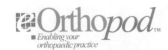

speeds up the degeneration. Scientists have also found links among family members, showing that genetics plays a role in how fast these changes occur.

Types of Pain

To help you understand the cause of your pain, spine specialists sometimes divide low back pain into two categories:

- Mechanical pain
- Neurogenic pain

Mechanical Pain

Mechanical pain is caused by wear and tear in the parts of the lumbar spine. Think of it like a machine that is wearing out. Mechanical pain usually starts from degenerative changes in the disc. As the disc begins to collapse and the space between the vertebrae narrows, the facet joints may become inflamed.

Mechanical pain tends to worsen with activity and ease with rest. It is usually felt in the low back but may spread into the buttocks, hips, and thighs. The pain rarely goes down past the knee. It usually doesn't cause weakness or numbness in the leg or foot because the problem is not from pressure on the spinal nerves.

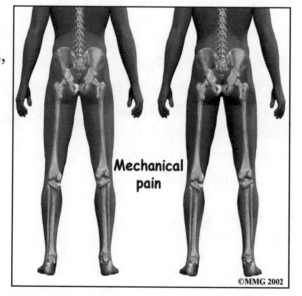

Mechanical pain

©MMG 2002

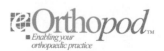
Enabling your orthopaedic practice

Back Care Boot Camp™

Notes

Neurogenic Pain

Neurogenic pain means "pain from nerve injury." Neurogenic pain occurs when spinal nerves are inflamed, squeezed, or pinched. A herniated disc or pinched nerve where it leaves the spine can cause this type of pain. We've also found that, when a disc ruptures, chemicals are released that can inflame the nerves, even if there is no pressure directly on them. Neurogenic pain is more concerning to healthcare providers than mechanical pain because it can damage the nerves and lead to weakness and numbness in the legs.

Pressure, inflammation, and irritation can affect the spinal nerve and cause symptoms in the areas where the nerve travels, rather than in the low back. The problem nerve affects structures away from the spine, such as the skin, joints, or muscles controlled by the nerve. As a result, your back may not hurt, yet you could feel pain, numbness, or weakness in your leg or foot. This indicates there's a problem in the body's electrical wiring. Muscles weaken. Reflexes slow. Sensations of pins, needles, and numbness may be felt where the nerve travels.

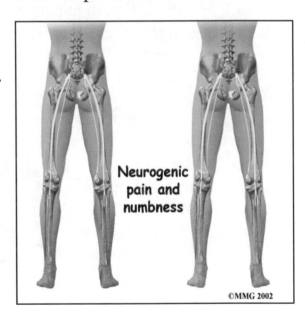

Neurogenic pain and numbness

©MMG 2002

Skills to Master

Over the past few visits, you've been practicing healthy posture, body mechanics, and lifting techniques. The strategies listed in this section are designed to get you thinking about ways to apply what you know in a variety of situations. In this session, you'll also learn how to calculate

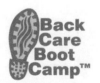

Back Care Boot Camp™

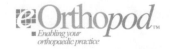

your aerobic exercise intensity. Perform only the items recommended by your doctor or therapist.

Posture Strategies

Driving

Rationale

Sitting puts a lot of pressure on the discs of the back. Driving in a car compounds the problem. Proper sitting postures can help you stay comfortable and protect your back while driving.

Description

Adjust the seat in your vehicle close enough so that your knees are bent and slightly higher than your hips. If your seat has an adjustable lumbar rest, set it so that it forms a slight inward curve in your low back. If you don't have 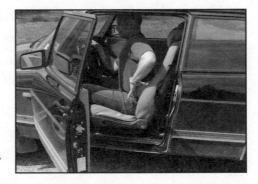 an adjustable lumbar support, you can roll up a towel and place it in the small of your low back.

Recommendations

Your doctor or therapist may suggest a lumbar roll or lumbar pillow to place in the small of your back when sitting and driving in a vehicle.

Concerns

Keeping your back in one position for a long time takes a toll on the health of your spine. You may find it helpful to routinely change the position of your low back on long drives. Do this by occasionally altering the setting of your lumbar support or by removing the towel, roll, or pillow from behind your back. Also, plan to stop at least every

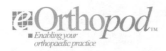
Enabling your orthopaedic practice

Notes

hour on long trips. Find a safe place to stop so you can get out of your vehicle and walk, stretch, and breathe.

Working at a Computer

Rationale

People who sit in front of a computer for long hours are at risk of back pain. Using safe postures and safe work strategies can improve comfort and protect your spine.

Description

Use a comfortable chair that supports your low back. Your shoulders should be relaxed, and your elbows, hips, and knees should be bent at right angles (90 degrees). Your feet should be flat on the floor or on a footrest. You can add support for your low back by rolling up a towel and placing it in the small of your low back.

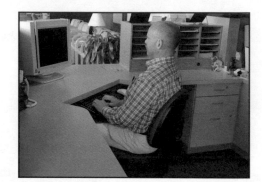

Recommendations

Your doctor or therapist may suggest a lumbar roll or lumbar pillow to support your low back in its neutral position while you work at a computer.

Concerns

Adjust the chair to support the slight inward curve of your low back. Avoid slouching by keeping the curve of your low back against the chair. Organize your work space so you can easily reach the items you use often. Make sure the work surface is the right height. If it's too high, you'll end up leaning forward with your arms stretched out instead of relaxed along your side. Be sure to take a break every 30 to 60 minutes to relax, breathe, and stretch.

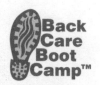

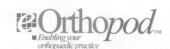

Lifting Strategies

We are constantly faced with the need to lift items. There are a variety of lifting styles that may prove useful at different times. Practice and use the choices listed here. Your therapist may determine that one style works best for you in most situations.

Lifting from a Car Trunk

Rationale

Lifting items out of a car trunk challenges the "rules of lifting." The bumper prevents you from bending your knees to lift. One way around this is to bend over at your waist and reach down to retrieve the item. But this can put your back in an unsafe position to lift. Protect your spine when lifting items out of the trunk by supporting your legs and by positioning your back in the power position.

Description

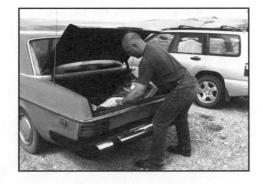

In situations where it is impossible to bend your knees to lift, you need to take special precautions. Get as close to the item as possible by supporting your knees against the car bumper. Bend at your hips, keeping your low back in the power position. Grasp the item firmly, and lift by extending your hips while keeping the slight inward curve in your low back. For heavier items, you may need to start by placing your knee on the bumper or the rim of the car trunk. Lean forward by bending your hips. Gather the item to your waist or onto your upper thigh. Then lift the item out of the trunk using your hip muscles. Keep your back in the neutral spine position.

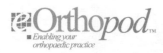

Notes

Recommendations

You need strong hip and back muscles to perform this lift safely. Your therapist can design exercises to help you strengthen these muscles.

Concerns

Getting a heavy item out of the trunk of a car can challenge safe lifting practices. So think twice before loading a heavy item into the trunk of your car. If you must get an item from the car trunk, only do it by yourself if you can keep your back in the power position. If not, get help.

Loading and Unloading a Dishwasher

Rationale

Repeated actions of bending and twisting the spine can hurt your back. Take every effort to move and lift safely when you load or unload a dishwasher. You can protect your back during this activity by bending with your hips and by pivoting with your feet.

Description

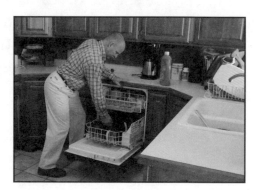

Face the dishwasher each time you reach to load or unload dishes. Bend from your hips, not your low back. Pivot your feet in the direction you are moving, rather than twisting with your back.

Recommendations

You may tend to bend over from your back if your leg muscles are weak. Your therapist can work with you to strengthen your buttock, hip, and thigh muscles.

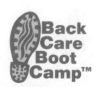

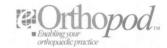

Concerns

Always position your back safely during this activity. Open and close the dishwasher door by bending with your hips and knees—not your back. It's easy to get in a rush and use poor habit when loading and unloading the dishwasher. Rely on your leg muscles. And keep from twisting your back by pivoting your feet.

Body Mechanic Strategies

Sweeping and Mopping

Rationale

It's hard to keep your back safely positioned while sweeping and mopping. You may tend to twist and flex your back to get the job done. But flexing and twisting your back at the same time is hazardous to the spine. The key is to engage your core muscles and to generate power from your hip and leg muscles. Practicing good technique may seem awkward at first, but it helps protect your back during these routine tasks.

Description

Keep your back in the power position, and engage your core muscles. You'll have better leverage as you work the broom or mop. If you need to lower yourself down to get under objects or to reach into tight spots, hinge at your hips so you keep from rounding your low back. Even small jobs should be done with care. Concentrate on engaging your core muscles and limiting how much you bend and twist your spine. Keep one leg forward when possible. Lean forward on your front leg with each stroke of the broom or mop. This focuses the action to your hips and legs—not your back.

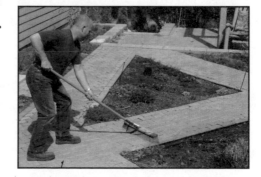

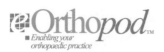
■ *Enabling your orthopaedic practice*

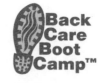
Back Care Boot Camp™

Notes

Recommendations

Practice engaging your core muscles and using your arms and legs to sweep or mop. You may be shown a partial lunge exercise to simulate the actions needed to complete these tasks safely.

Concerns

Avoid the tendency to twist from side to side when sweeping or mopping. And don't twist or bend your trunk to get under objects or to reach into tight spots. If you don't engage your core muscles, you'll be forced to flex and twist your back. Be cautious when using a dust pan or mop bucket. Remember to bend with your hips and knees rather than keeping your legs straight, which forces you to bend at your waist.

Vacuuming

Rationale

People with back pain often have difficulty vacuuming. Poor technique takes a toll on the long-term health of the spine and actually requires more energy than using good technique. As when sweeping and mopping, you may find it awkward at first to keep your back safely positioned while vacuuming. But by using your core muscles and by generating power from your hips and legs, you'll protect your back. And you'll need less energy than when you use only your arms to push and pull the vacuum.

Description

Keep your back in the power position, and engage your core muscles. You'll have better leverage as you work the vacuum back and forth. When you push the vacuum forward, keep one leg in front of the other, and lean forward on your

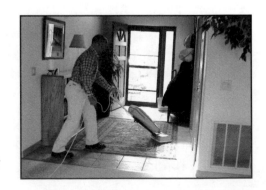

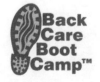

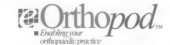

Notes

front leg. Then lean back onto your back leg as you pull the vacuum toward you. This focuses the action to your hips and legs—not your back. If you need to lower yourself down to get under objects or to reach into tight spots, hinge at your hips to keep from rounding your low back. You might find it easiest to get down onto one knee in these situations.

Recommendations

Practice engaging your core and using your hip and leg muscles as you vacuum. You may be shown a partial lunge exercise to simulate the actions needed to complete this task safely.

Concerns

Keep the vacuum directly in front of you at all times. Avoid trying to reach around corners or objects. This will force you to bend and twist your low back. Don't twist or bend your trunk to get under objects or to reach into tight spots. Use the rules of safe lifting (described in Session Four) when lifting and transporting the vacuum.

Exercises

Follow your therapist's guidance about the types of exercises you do. Continue your daily stretching routine. As you build strength and control in your core muscles, use this new and improved strength as you go about your daily activities.

Aerobic Conditioning

Continue to step up your aerobic exercise program. People who stay active and improve their cardiovascular fitness tend to get better, faster. Aerobic exercise also helps people cope with back pain.

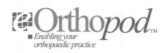

Notes

Calculating Intensity

Rationale

You've been gradually increasing the amount of time (duration) you spend on your aerobic workout. Now it's time to increase the *intensity* of your exercise. Intensity is how hard you work during exercise. Knowing ways to calculate the intensity of your workout can ensure that you don't overdo it. It also provides a starting point for setting exercise goals.

Description

You can monitor your heart rate to know how hard you're working out. The easiest way to do this is by wearing a heart-rate monitor, which shows your heart's beats per minute (bpm). You can also check your heart rate without a special device by taking your pulse. To take your pulse, place the pad of one finger lightly over the front of the opposite wrist, just below the thumb. Count the pulses for 15 seconds and multiply them by four. (For example, 20 pulses in 15 seconds is 80 bpm.) You'll use this number to track how hard you're working out. If you're not able to feel your pulse at your wrist, you can place the two pads of fingers on the carotid artery, located on the side of your neck.

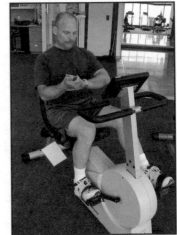

To target the intensity of your workout, obtain your maximum heart rate (MHR) by subtracting your age

Calculating an Exercise Target

For a 50-year-old woman, the equation for MHR looks like this: 220 − 50 = 170 bpm.

Her MHR is 170 bpm. She multiplies her MHR by the intensity target. If we assume she's physically fit, she could multiply her MHR by 80 percent.

170 x .8 = 136 bpm

So during her exercise routine, she should feel 34 pulses when checking her pulse for 15 seconds. It looks like this: 34 x 4 = 136 bpm.

Back Care Boot Camp™

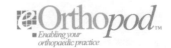

Ortho*pod*™
Enabling your orthopaedic practice

from 220. Then multiply by a percentage between 50 and 85 percent. If you're just starting out, shoot for 50 to 60 percent of your MHR. Eventually you can progress toward a high-energy workout by targeting between 75 and 85 percent. (Refer to the target heart rate example for calculating an exercise target.)

Another way to check how hard you're working is to rate how you feel when you're working out. This method uses a rate of perceived exertion (RPE) scale. While exercising, choose a number between zero and 10, where one means you're hardly doing anything (no exertion), and 10 means you're at your maximum exertion. Shoot for an RPE between four and six. Your RPE represents the amount of work you feel in your muscles and how hard you're breathing.

Recommendations

Your doctor or therapist will help you determine your exercise heart rate. Check your pulse often at first while exercising to check that you are meeting your intensity target. Also, rate your intensity from zero to 10 (your RPE) and track it when you check your heart rate. Your RPE should equate closely to your exercise heart rate. In other words, at 60 percent of your maximum heart rate, you may feel that you're working with an RPE of five. Advancing to 80 percent of your maximum heart rate will cause your RPE to rise, perhaps to a seven or eight.

After a while, you may find that you only need to keep an eye on your RPE, as it will give you a good idea about what your heart rate is doing. Use your current exercise levels to set goals. Goals can help make your aerobic exercise program meaningful and fun.

Concerns

Beginners, sedentary people, and older patients should target between 50 and 60 percent of their

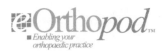

Notes

maximum heart rate. This percentage can safely go up as your body adjusts to a longer workout with greater intensity. Check with your doctor or therapist if you have problems tracking the intensity of your aerobic workout.

Drill Time

Practice the skills and exercises shown by your therapist in this session. You'll be asked to demonstrate them during your next clinic visit. If you have pain or problems while practicing, your therapist can help at your next Drill Time.

Demonstrate

You may have been shown some or all of the items listed below. Go over them with your therapist to make sure you're doing them safely and correctly.

Practice Lifting

- Ball squat
- Mock lift

Lifting Styles

- Golfer's lift
- Diagonal lift
- Power lift

Lifting Strategies

- Lifting infants and kids
- Loading and unloading a clothes dryer

Exercise

- Core stabilization exercises
- Home exercise program

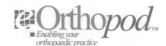

Practice

Use this list as a reminder of the skills and exercises you'll be practicing. Practice only the skills and exercises demonstrated by your therapist. Don't create your own exercises or go on to the next level without talking to your therapist.

Posture Strategies

- Driving
- Working at a computer

Lifting Strategies

- Lifting from a car trunk
- Loading and unloading a dishwasher

Body Mechanic Strategies

- Sweeping
- Mopping
- Vacuuming

Exercise

- Taking your heart rate
- Calculating your target heart rate
- Calculating your rate of perceived exertion (RPE)

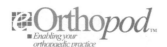

Notes

Questions for Review

1. How would you describe the degenerative model of back pain?

2. How can degenerative changes in the spine cause back pain and problems?

3. How do mechanical pain and neurogenic pain differ?

Think about these questions. They will be reviewed at the start of your next session.

Session Review

The degenerative model of back pain describes a chain reaction of changes.

- At first the nucleus weakens, tears, and scars.

- As disc height decreases, the vertebrae move closer together.

- This puts pressure on the facet joints, which can cause them to become arthritic.

- Changes in the ligaments, discs, and facet joints can cause the spinal segment to become loose and unstable.

- Bone spurs form on the vertebrae.

- The nucleus may squeeze (herniate) through the weakened annulus

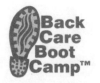

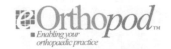
Enabling your orthopaedic practice

Mechanical pain comes from wear and tear on the parts of the spine.

- It's like a machine that is wearing out.

- It usually gets worse with activity and eases with rest.

- The pain rarely goes down past the knee.

- It usually doesn't cause weakness or numbness.

Neurogenic pain comes from a nerve injury.

- It occurs when spinal nerves are inflamed, squeezed, or pinched.

- It can cause pain and symptoms that affect structures away from the spine.

Neurogenic pain is more concerning than mechanical pain.

- Neurogenic pain involves the spinal nerves and can lead to weakness and numbness in the legs.

- Mechanical pain usually doesn't affect the nerves.

Protect your back while sweeping and mopping.

- Engage your core muscles to keep you from twisting back and forth.

- Keep one leg in front of the other and lean forward and back from your hips.

Sample calculations of the training heart rate for a sedentary 40-year-old man.

- 220 − 40 = 180 (180 is his maximum heart rate).

- 180 x .6 = 104 beats per minute (bpm).

- He should feel 26 pulses in 15 seconds during exercises (26 x 4 = 104 bpm).

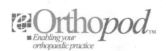

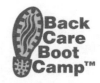

Notes

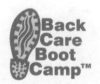
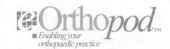

Session Six: Master Your Back Program

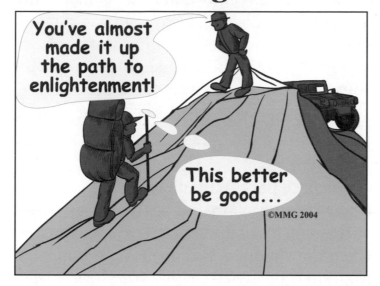

Goals for This Session

- Define *nonspecific low back pain.*

- Explain the usual course of first-time low back pain.

- List three parts of the spine that can be a source of low back pain.

- Relate your knowledge of anatomy to various spine conditions.

- Define "red flags" for actively seeking medical help.

- Begin to engage the relaxation response.

- Demonstrate mastery of your back program.

Information to Master

It's time for a little celebration. You've cleared the half-way point in *Back Care Boot Camp* and are nearing completion of the program. This session is devoted to helping you master your back program. If you have any questions about the information and skills you've been gathering since Session One, take the time now to discuss them with your doctor or therapist.

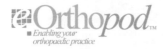

Enabling your orthopaedic practice

Notes

You learned early in the program simple ways to take care of your back pain by applying heat or ice, by positioning your back for comfort, and by using healthy back postures. You began exercises to help you move and function easier. And you learned the importance of using your core muscles during activities like lifting to protect your back from further pain and injury.

You'll find in this session that most back pain usually goes away quickly. Unfortunately, most people who have back pain once will have it again. Scientists estimate that as many as 90 percent of back patients will have recurring back pain, which returns again and again. That's why it is so important that you learn and apply ways of controlling symptoms when they happen. But even more importantly, your back program is designed to give you the knowledge, exercises, skills, and resources to improve your chances of avoiding recurring back pain.

Most people who have first-time back pain get better in a matter of days or weeks. They usually don't need any special or sophisticated tests (such as X-rays or MRI scans) unless concerns, or "red flags," are raised. Later in this session you'll learn what these red flags are and what should be done if they appear. In rare cases, specialized medical tests may be needed, along with further treatments, if symptoms don't go away as expected.

Before jumping ahead, spend time recalling what you learned in Session Five. Review the answers to last session's Questions for Review.

Answers for Review

In the last session, you were asked three questions. Take a few moments to compare your answers to those given here.

1. How would you describe the degenerative model of back pain?

Most back problems are from wear and tear on the parts of the spine over many years. This process is called *degeneration*.

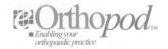

Notes

Over time, the normal process of aging can result in degenerative changes in all parts of the spine. These are natural changes that happen with the passing of time. Some people experience pain from these changes; others don't.

2. How can degenerative changes in the spine cause back pain and problems?

At first, the annulus weakens, tears, and scars. Cracks in the outer part of the annulus can cause pain. The nucleus loses water content, leading to a decrease in disc height. As the vertebrae move closer together, the facet joints are compressed and can become arthritic. Changes in the ligaments, discs, and facet joints can cause the spinal segment to become loose and unstable. The nucleus may squeeze (herniate) through the weakened annulus. Pain can occur when the disc puts pressure on nearby spinal nerve roots and when the damaged nucleus emits pain-causing chemicals.

3. How do mechanical pain and neurogenic pain differ?

Mechanical back pain is caused by wear and tear in the parts of the lumbar spine. It typically gets worse after activity and is usually felt in the back, buttocks, hips, and thighs. It is less concerning than *neurogenic pain* because it doesn't involve nerve problems. Neurogenic pain comes from nerve injury. The irritated nerve causes symptoms in the areas where the nerve travels, rather than in the low back. The irritated nerve affects how the body functions. Muscles weaken. Reflexes slow. Sensations of pins, needles, and numbness may be felt where the nerve travels.

Getting Specific about "Nonspecific" Low Back Pain

Back pain is rarely life-threatening, and it's usually not from a serious disease. In fact, most people who have back pain for the first time get better in a matter of a few days to several weeks. So relax! And breathe deeply. By doing so, you'll be on track to master your back pain.

When back pain first occurs, the pain can set you back for a short time. At first, you might even need to take a break from activities for a short while. But as you learned in Session One, it's generally a good idea to get back to daily and work activities sooner rather than later.

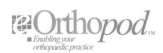

Notes

Many people who have a first go-round of back pain will have back pain again within a couple of years. Still, the problem isn't necessarily serious, and people can generally return to normal activity in a short amount of time. But just because your back pain isn't serious doesn't mean you should ignore it. It is important to try and understand it.

Most often, back pain is a mechanical problem. As you learned in the last session, mechanical back pain tends to occur with activity and go away with rest. Although it starts in the low back, you may feel it spread into one or both buttocks. It rarely goes down past the back of the knee. Your back may feel stiff in the morning, and your pain may feel worse as the day goes on.

The first time this type of back pain strikes, your doctor may refer to it as "simple" or "nonspecific" back pain. You may think the pain is anything but simple! However, you need to understand that this type of problem is not serious. It simply means your back isn't moving and working normally. You haven't damaged your back. Your doctor probably won't need to run any special or high-tech tests to figure out what's going on. Hopefully all you need is reassurance that you're going to be okay. With *Back Care Boot Camp*, you are learning how to take care of problems if and when they arise.

You can learn to understand your back pain better. First you need to learn about areas of the spine that can register pain. Pain is a sensation, just like touch and pressure are sensations. To feel sensations like pain, our body has special receptors, or sensors, that signal our nervous system. There are several structures in the back that have sensors to register pain. Refer to the chart below to see which parts of the spine can be a source of back pain.

Making "Sense" of Back Pain

- **Muscle:** Muscles rarely send pain information, but the tendons on the ends of muscles may register pain.

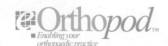

- **Bone:** The covering around bones, called the *periosteum*, has sensors for pain.

- **Disc:** The outer portion of the annulus can register pain, especially when a crack forms in this area.

- **Ligament:** These supportive tissues have many pain sensors.

- **Nerve:** Irritation of the sheath around the spinal nerve can register pain or other symptoms.

- **Joint:** The enclosure of a joint, called the *capsule*, is richly supplied with pain sensors.

You can see from this list that back pain can begin in many parts of the spine. The main goal when treating nonspecific back pain is to help you get moving and avoid disabling pain. It's not as important for your healthcare provider to figure out exactly which structures in your back are registering pain.

Spine Conditions

In Session Five, you learned about the changes that sometimes happen in the spine over time. These degenerative changes seem to occur in just about everyone, but only some people end up feeling back pain. Degenerative changes can sometimes lead to certain spine conditions. The conditions listed here represent some of the conditions that spine experts know about.

- Annular tears
- Internal disc disruption
- Herniated disc
- Facet joint arthritis
- Segmental instability
- Spinal stenosis
- Foraminal stenosis

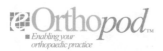

Annular Tears

As you know by now, our intervertebral discs change with age, much like our hair turns gray. Perhaps the earliest stage of degeneration occurs due to tears that occur in the annulus. These tears can result from wear and tear over a period of time. They can also be the result of a sudden injury to the disc, such as a twist, or an increased strain that overpowers the strength of the annulus. These annular tears may cause back pain until they heal with scar tissue.

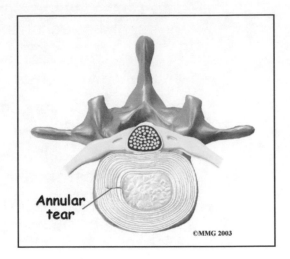

Annular tear

©MMG 2003

Internal Disc Disruption

Multiple annular tears can lead to a weakened disc. The disc starts to degenerate and collapse. The vertebrae begin to compress. The collapsing disc can be the source of pain because it has lost the ability to be a shock absorber between the vertebrae. This condition is sometimes referred to as *internal disc disruption*. This type of problem causes primarily mechanical back pain due to inflammation of the disc and surrounding structures.

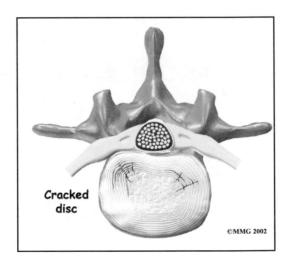

Cracked disc

©MMG 2002

Herniated Disc

A disc that has been weakened may rupture, or herniate. If the annulus ruptures, or tears, the material in the nucleus can squeeze out of the disc, or herniate. A disc herniation usually causes neurogenic pain if the disc presses against a spinal nerve. The chemicals released by the disc may also

Back Care Boot Camp™

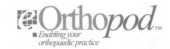
Enabling your orthopaedic practice

inflame the nerve root, causing pain in the area where the nerve travels down the leg. This type of leg pain is called *sciatica*.

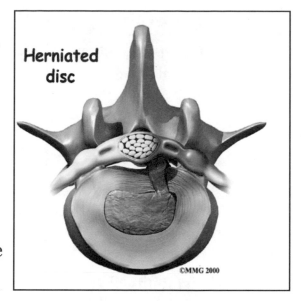

Herniated disc

©MMG 2000

Even a normal disc can rupture. Heavy, repetitive bending, twisting, and lifting can place too much pressure on the disc, causing the annulus to tear and the nucleus to rupture into the spinal canal.

Facet Joint Arthritis

The facet joints along the back of the spinal column link the vertebrae together. They are not meant to bear much weight. However, if a disc loses its height, the vertebra above the disc begins to press down on the vertebra below. This causes the facet joints to press together. Articular cartilage covers the surfaces where these joints meet. Like other joints in the body that are covered with articular cartilage, the facet joints can develop *osteoarthritis* as the articular cartilage wears away over time. Extra pressure on the facet joints,

such as that caused by a collapsing disc, can speed the degeneration in the facet joints. The swelling and inflammation from an arthritic facet joint can be a source of low back pain.

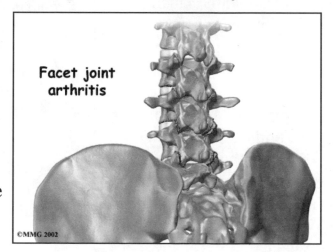

Facet joint arthritis

©MMG 2002

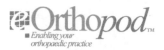
Orthopod™
■ *Enabling your orthopaedic practice*

Back Care Boot Camp™

Notes

Segmental Instability

Segmental instability means that the vertebral bones within a spinal segment move more than they should. Instability can develop in the low back if a disc has degenerated. Usually the supporting ligaments around the problem vertebrae have also been stretched over time.

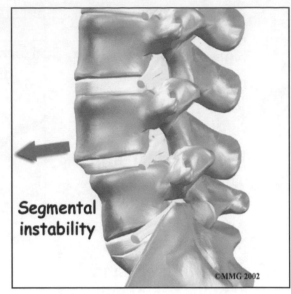

Segmental instability

©MMG 2002

Segmental instability also includes conditions in which a vertebral body begins to slip over the one below it. When a vertebral body slips too far forward, the condition is called *spondylolisthesis*. Whatever the cause, this extra movement in the bones of the spine can create problems. It can lead to mechanical pain simply because the structures of the spine move around too much and become inflamed and painful. The extra movement can also cause neurogenic pain if the spinal nerves are squeezed as a result of the segmental instability.

Spinal Stenosis

Stenosis means "closing in." *Spinal stenosis* refers to a condition in which the tissues inside the spinal canal are "closed in," or compressed. The spinal cord ends at L2. Below this level, the spinal canal contains spinal nerves that travel to the pelvis and legs. When stenosis narrows the spinal canal in the low back, the spinal nerves can be squeezed inside the canal.

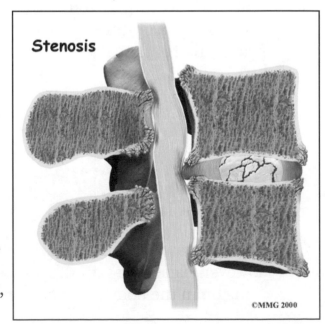

Stenosis

©MMG 2000

Back Care Boot Camp™

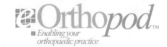

Orthopod™
Enabling your orthopaedic practice

The pressure from the spinal stenosis can cause problems in the way the nerves work. The resulting problems include pain and numbness in the buttocks and legs and weakness in the muscles served by the nerves. Pressure on the nerves that go to the bladder and rectum is a cause for concern because it can weaken the muscles that control the bladder and bowels.

Foraminal Stenosis

Spinal nerves exit the spinal canal between the vertebrae in a tunnel called the *neural foramen*. Anything that causes this tunnel to become smaller can squeeze the spinal nerve as it passes through the tunnel. This condition is called *foraminal stenosis*, meaning that the foramen is narrowed. As the disc collapses and loses height through degeneration, the vertebral body above begins to collapse toward the one below. The opening around the spinal nerve narrows,

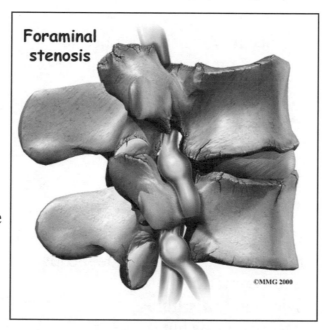

Foraminal stenosis

©MMG 2000

squeezing the nerve. Arthritis of the facet joints can cause bone spurs to form and point into the foramen, causing further nerve compression and irritation. Foraminal stenosis can cause a combination of mechanical and neurogenic pain.

Raising a Red Flag

Back pain is not a disease, and symptoms of back pain usually go away in a matter of days or weeks. In rare cases, however, back pain can be a signal that something else is going on in the body. Your doctor and therapist likely asked

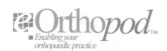

Notes

many questions at first about your symptoms and general health. They were checking to make sure there were no "red flags" that would alert them to other possible causes of your pain (such as kidney stones, infection, or cancer). The box on the right lists some of these red flags.

You should also know of other concerning symptoms that require immediate attention. If these occur, you need to "raise a red flag" for prompt medical attention.

- Cauda equina syndrome
- Worsening leg numbness or weakness
- Worsening pain

Cauda Equina Syndrome

The *cauda equina*, which is Latin for "horse's tail," is the bundle of nerve fibers inside the lower spinal canal that radiate out to the trunk, pelvis, and lower limbs. Pressure on this bundle of nerves causes distinctive symptoms including low back pain, pain running down the back of both legs, and numbness or tingling between the legs in the area you would contact if you were seated on a saddle. The pressure can disturb function of the bowels and bladder. You need

Red Flag Circumstances

- Bad trauma
- Mid-back pain
- Changes in bowel or bladder function
- Back pain with no apparent cause
- Back pain in a person under 20 or over 55 years old
- Severe night pain
- Symptoms unaltered by body position
- A previous diagnosis of cancer
- Recent and significant weight loss

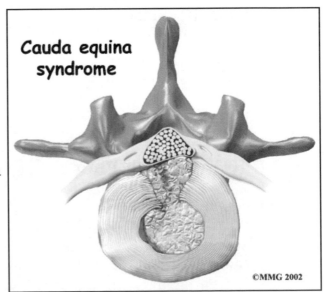

Cauda equina syndrome

©MMG 2002

Back Care Boot Camp™

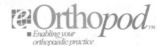

Orthopod™

■ *Enabling your orthopaedic practice*

Notes

to raise a flag if you feel the need to urinate, but can't, or if you lose bowel or bladder control. Cauda equina syndrome is an emergency. If the pressure isn't relieved, it can lead to permanent paralysis of the bowels and bladder. Doctors usually recommend immediate surgery to remove pressure from the nerves.

Worsening Leg Numbness or Weakness

You should also alert your healthcare provider if you feel leg weakness or numbness that is steadily getting worse. These symptoms may signal increasing pressure on the nerves going to your lower limbs.

Worsening Pain

The third red flag is not as crucial as the previous two. But a flag should be raised if you feel significant back or leg pain that seems only to be getting worse. In this case, it is time to regroup with your doctor to pursue other tests and treatments.

Skills to Master

You are in the final sessions of *Back Care Boot Camp*. The focus of this session is on mastering your back program, which starts with your state of mind. That's right! In order to master your back program, you need to master your mind. How are you responding to your back pain? Have you resumed normal activity? Are you fearful?

Stop for a moment. Do you realize that the major factor in disabling back pain is fear? Fear is actually dangerous, especially if you are fearful that you'll hurt yourself again, that you won't get better, or that you won't get back to normal living. The way you respond to your situation can be more disabling than back pain itself.

Realize that you've gained knowledge that can help you combat this downward spiral. You've learned that most episodes of back pain are short-lived, are not serious or life-threatening, and are manageable. So relax. And breathe.

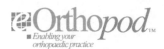

Literally! This is precisely where mastering your back begins. In this skills section, you'll gain tools to change the way you think about your back pain—skills that will help you gain control, change your mindset, and employ the discipline you'll need to master your back program!

Relax Your Mind and Body

Take a moment right now and analyze yourself. Are you anxious and tense? Or are you relaxed and happy? Stress from back pain can throw you off and alter your focus. Your response to your situation matters. It can make the difference between taking control of your back pain, or having back pain take control of you. The relaxation response can help.

Engage the Relaxation Response

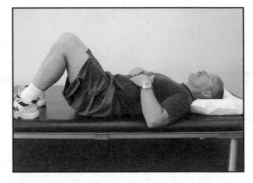

By engaging the relaxation response, you change the way you think. You begin to regain control and the focus you need to successfully master your back program. Only you can take charge. You must decide to stop and get focused. Until you do, you won't get the full benefit from all the other information you've learned in *Back Care Boot Camp* to help you take care of your back. So stop right now. Regain your focus. Engage the relaxation response.

Rationale

The relaxation response is a skill for your body and mind. By combining healthy breathing and calm thoughts in a relaxing atmosphere, your body and mind both benefit. Your body benefits because muscles relax, blood pressure drops, and pain eases. Your mind benefits because stress

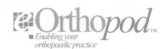

calms, focus clears, and thoughts become streamlined. When you engage the relaxation response, you'll be in a frame of mind that enables you to deal with your situation and successfully apply all the other helpful skills you've learned to help you master your back.

Description

There are many ways to engage the relaxation response. Most involve one to two daily sessions of relaxed breathing and focused thinking in calm surroundings. It's a simple, nearly effortless way to allow your body a few moments to unwind. As you relax the body, you relax the mind. This form of meditation doesn't require a big change in your beliefs. It is not religious and requires only a small time commitment. Follow these steps to engage the relaxation response:

• Choose a word, phrase, or prayer to focus on.

• Get comfortable—wherever you are. If you're at home, you could sit in your favorite chair. You may prefer to lie down in a comfortable position.

• Use your diaphragm to breathe. Feel your abdomen rise and fall rhythmically.

• Recite your word, phrase, or prayer with each breath you take.

• Begin to relax your muscles one by one, starting with your toes and feet, and then your lower legs. Slowly work your way muscle by muscle to the top of your head.

• Ignore worries, deadlines, fears, and thoughts about the day.

• Continue for 10 to 20 minutes.

• Collect your thoughts. Allow new and focused thoughts to gain a foothold before you rise and go about your daily tasks.

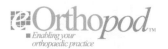

Notes

Recommendations

Find a model of relaxation that fits your beliefs. There are many resources available to assist you. Session Eight provides a brief overview of some options. Talk further with your doctor or therapist for other helpful ideas.

Concerns

People who don't engage the relaxation response may miss the full benefit of all the skills in *Back Care Boot Camp*. If you don't take the time and effort to gain control of your situation, these other tools lose some of their effectiveness.

Plan for the Future

The outlook is positive for a healthy back. Even if back pain should someday strike again, which it might, you know

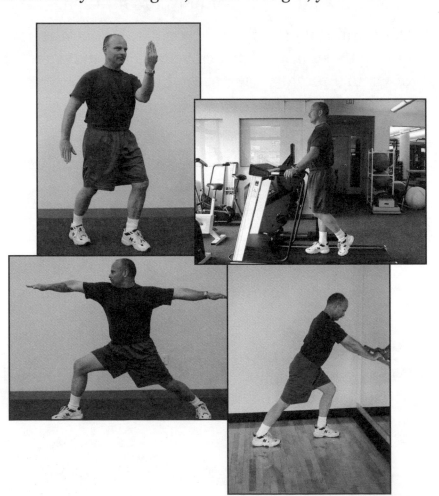

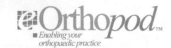

what to do and the steps to take. The information and skills you've learned are designed to reduce your chances of future pain and problems. Mastering your back program requires making a plan for the future. Are you planning to stop smoking? Will you begin a fitness program? Should you join a health club? Begin developing your plan now. You'll need to complete it by the time you finish *Back Care Boot Camp*.

Making a Plan

Rationale

Taking care of your back is your business. Make it your business by creating a workable plan, one that will keep you moving toward improved spine health. By picking a routine that fits your lifestyle, chances are good that you'll stick with your routine.

Description

A lifelong approach to spine health should center on activities you enjoy. There are many activity choices— everything from support groups and yoga to water therapy and personal training. Start by learning about all the resources available. Pick an activity you enjoy. Ideally, you'll be able to locate programs and services near you. You can identify them by consulting the health section of your local newspaper, by looking in the phone book, and by talking with your doctor and therapist.

Recommendations

Use the form called *Making a Plan* to help you narrow down your choices and to establish your future plan. Present your completed plan to your therapist during your last session. By doing so, you will have demonstrated mastery of your back program, and you will be ready to graduate from *Back Care Boot Camp*.

Concerns

You've gained momentum to this point in *Back Care Boot Camp*. By not crafting a workable plan, this momentum

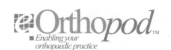

will stop. You may even limit your options for a healthier tomorrow. The key to keeping your back healthy is to participate in an ongoing and active routine, one that you enjoy and that will keep your interests for the years ahead.

Drill Time

Practice the skills and exercises shown by your therapist in this session. You'll be asked to demonstrate them during your next clinic visit. If you have pain or problems while practicing, your therapist can help at your next Drill Time.

Demonstrate

You may have been shown some or all of the items listed below. Go over them with your therapist to make sure you're doing them safely and correctly.

Posture Strategies

- Driving
- Working at a computer

Lifting Strategies

- Lifting from a car trunk
- Loading and unloading a dishwasher

Body Mechanic Strategies

- Sweeping
- Mopping
- Vacuuming

Exercise

- Taking your exercise heart rate
- Calculating your target heart rate
- Calculating your rate of perceived exertion (RPE)
- Home exercise program

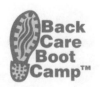
Back Care Boot Camp™

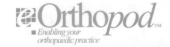
Enabling your orthopaedic practice

Practice

Use this list as a reminder of the skills and exercises you'll be practicing. Practice only the skills and exercises demonstrated by your therapist. Don't create your own exercises or go on to the next level without talking to your therapist.

Engaging the Relaxation Response

- Breathing
- Relaxing
- Meditating
- Focusing

Making a Plan

- Identify ways to actively pursue lifelong spine health.
- Find programs and services in your location.
- Complete the form called *Making a Plan*.

Questions for Review

1. How would you describe nonspecific low back pain?

2. Which spine structures can be a source of low back pain?

3. When should a person with back pain raise a "red flag" for prompt medical attention?

Think about these questions. They will be reviewed at the start of your next session.

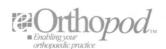
Enabling your
orthopaedic practice

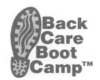

Notes

Session Review

Nonspecific back pain usually goes away in time.

- It's not a disease and is not life-threatening.

- Most people with first-time back pain get better within a few days to several weeks.

- Their problem is usually mechanical, meaning that their back isn't working right.

- They rarely need special tests to figure out what's going on.

- Resuming activity swiftly is more important than knowing the exact source of pain.

- Nine of 10 people who have back pain once will have back pain that recurs.

There are steps you can take when back pain strikes.

- Apply heat or ice to the sore area.

- Position your back for comfort.

- Use postures that take pressure off the sore area.

- Get moving sooner rather than later.

You can take steps to avoid future back pain.

- Develop and use core muscles, especially with tasks like lifting.

- Use proper posture, body mechanics, and lifting techniques.

- Avoid tobacco.

- Maintain reasonable body weight.

- Stay flexible and conditioned.

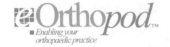

Several structures in the spine can be a source of back pain.

- Muscle: Muscles rarely cause pain, but tendons attaching on the ends can register pain.

- Bone: The periosteum (bone surface) has sensors for pain.

- Disc: The outer rings of the annulus sense pain, especially when cracks form in this area.

- Ligament: When these supportive structures are stretched or torn, they send pain signals.

- Nerve: The sheath that covers spinal nerves has sensors for pain.

- Joint: The capsule enclosing spinal joints is rich with pain sensors.

Degeneration leads to these conditions.

- Annular tears: Small tears in the outer ring of the disc commonly occur as part of the degenerative process. The tears can also come from sudden injury to the disc, such as a twist or strain that overpowers the strength of the annulus.

- Herniated disc: The nucleus in the center of the disc pushes through the annulus. A herniated nucleus can cause neurogenic pain. The chemicals released can inflame the nerve root, leading to sciatica (pain that travels down the leg in the area of the spinal nerve).

- Facet joint arthritis: Degeneration causes the disc to collapse and the facet joints to press together. The articular cartilage on the surface of the facet joints can become osteoarthritic, much like other joints in the body.

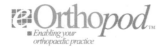
■ *Enabling your orthopaedic practice*

Notes

Three "red flags" need immediate medical attention.

- Cauda equina syndrome.

- Worsening leg numbness or weakness.

- Back or leg pain that is getting worse.

Your body and mind benefit from engaging the relaxation response.

- Your body benefits because muscles relax, blood pressure drops, and pain eases.

- Your mind benefits because stress calms, focus clears, and thoughts become streamlined.

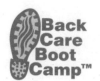

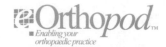

Session Seven: Back to Work

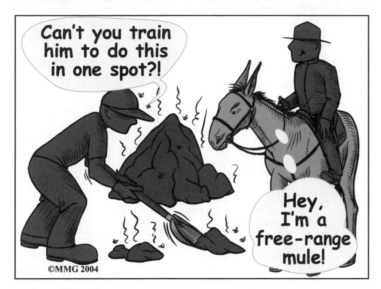

 ## Goals for This Session

- Know the parts of your job or activities that can affect your back.

- Discover factors that can influence work-related back pain.

- Know the barriers that can keep you from getting back to work or play.

- Learn how therapists team up to help manage back problems at work.

- Apply strategies to make your work, hobby, or home environment safer.

- Know what steps you can take to prevent back pain at work and play.

 ## Information to Master

Not everyone who works has back pain. And not everyone with back pain works. So whether you're trying to get safely back to work, recreation, or hobbies, you'll find helpful tips in this session. As you go through this session, you'll see many references to workers and the workplace.

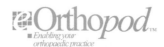
Enabling your orthopaedic practice

Notes

But similar principles may be applied when people are attempting to return safely to a particular sport, activity, or hobby.

The activities and work we do influence our chances of having back pain. Researchers are still trying to determine which activities pose the most risk for back trouble. Is it harder on your back to sit all day, or is it better to be on your feet? Does being sedentary at work pose greater problems than doing physically challenging work? Many questions remain unanswered.

It has been shown that people in jobs that require heavy lifting, bending, and twisting tend to report back symptoms and back injuries more often than people in less demanding jobs. Ironically, scientists believe that the risks from these heavy activities probably have a smaller role in back problems than other factors in workers' lives. Do the workers smoke heavily? Are they physically unfit? Do they routinely recreate or do hobbies that put an even bigger strain on the spine?

In this session, we'll look at these and other factors that may have a role in back problems at the workplace. But what about people who've had a back injury or experienced back pain at work? Today's advice is that if they are working, they should probably stay on the job. And those who are off work due to back problems should attempt to get back to work sooner, rather than later. Recall from Session One that people generally recover faster when they stay active and resume normal activities as soon as possible after having back pain or a back injury.

The longer people stay off work, the greater their risk for long-term pain and disability. And the longer they're off, the smaller the chance they'll get back to work. It is important that employees with back pain return to work as soon as they can, even if they're still feeling some pain. There are many good reasons why staying on the job is a good idea. People at work tend to stay more active. They

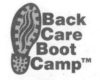
Back Care Boot Camp™

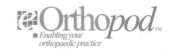

enjoy the social interaction of being at work. Their self-image is raised because they see themselves as productive workers. They sense that they are well, not "ill." And they find that their pain, though often annoying, is not disabling.

Sometimes there are barriers that keep people from getting back to the job. This session will look at these barriers and what people can do to overcome them as they attempt to get back to work.

Before jumping ahead, spend time recalling what you learned in Session Six. Review the answers to the last session's Questions for Review.

Answers for Review

In the last session, you were asked three questions. Take a few moments to compare your answers to those given here.

1. How would you describe nonspecific low back pain?

Nonspecific pain is the most common type of back pain. It's usually a signal that the back is not working right. The spine hasn't been damaged. The pain is "mechanical," and it usually goes away in a matter of a few days to several weeks. People do best when they use simple measures to take care of the pain and when they get moving sooner, rather than later.

2. Which spine structures can be a source of low back pain?

The spine has numerous structures that can be a source of low back pain. They include muscles, discs, bones, ligaments, joints, and nerves.

3. When should a person with back pain raise a "red flag" for prompt medical attention?

First, immediate attention is needed when symptoms of cauda equina syndrome occur. These symptoms can include back pain, pain going down the backs of one or both thighs, disturbed function of the bowels or bladder, and numbness in the genital area. Second, numbness or weakness in the lower limbs that is steadily getting worse requires prompt attention. And third, people who feel back or leg pain that continues to get worse should report their symptoms to their doctor and therapist.

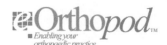

Notes

Connecting the Dots from Work to Back Pain

Back injuries are the most common work-related injury. They are one of the most frequent reasons for work absence. What is the connection between working and the onset of back pain? In industrialized nations where vast amounts of money are spent on work-related back pain, this is a multi-billion-dollar question. The connection isn't always clear. But today's research shows that numerous factors are at play, many of which probably work together as the real causes of back pain.

Obvious factors in back pain include smoking and obesity. If you smoke or are overweight, help is available so you can face these problems. By addressing these issues, you immediately improve your outlook for improved spine health. Talk to your healthcare provider for suggestions.

The physical demands of the job can also contribute to back pain among workers. Back injuries are more often reported by workers who have to deal with extremely heavy loads at work. As you'll recall from Session Four, lifting is often blamed as a cause of back pain. But lifting itself is not necessarily a risk factor for back pain until other variables are added. For example, lifting becomes a risk when poor technique is used, such as lifting when the back is bent and especially when it is twisted. People who must lift more than half of the work day or who must repeatedly lift 50 pounds or more are also at risk for work-related back pain. There is also some evidence that workers who are exposed to whole

Influences on Work-Related Back Pain

- Obesity

- Smoking

- Low job satisfaction

- Low education levels

- Working lots of overtime

- Sedentary work conditions

- No influence on work conditions

- Work that involves whole body vibration

- Driving more than one-half of the work day

- Dealing with extremely heavy loads at work

- A past episode of back pain or previous back injury

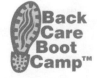

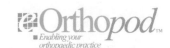

Notes

body vibration are at risk for back pain. Driving is the main culprit for this type of vibration. It is estimated that people who drive more than half their work day may be at greater risk of work-related back pain.

There is a connection between back pain and peoples' attitudes at work. Where there is high job satisfaction and good relationships throughout the company, there are generally fewer problems with back pain and back injuries. Stressful jobs and jobs where people don't feel they have any influence on what happens at work report more back problems.

Employers have a growing awareness about how they can help combat back problems at work. Many are beginning to work more closely with employees to identify problem areas, to encourage greater communication through the workforce, and to address potential problems. Developing this type of "safety culture" is showing modest results. Companies with this model in place sometimes see a drop in the reported number of back problems.

Jumping Hurdles to Get Back to Work

People with back pain sometimes run into barriers that keep them from returning to work. Being warned about these barriers can help you know ahead of time what to look out for and where you may need extra help. If you see barriers that may be holding you back, talk with your doctor and therapist. They will attempt to learn all they can about your job to help you work around any obstacles.

People who've injured their back while doing their job may be afraid of hurting themselves again. Their fear of re-injury strongly predicts that they'll have a harder time getting back to their jobs. Studies show that this type of fear accounts for about 25 percent of work disability. This means that in at least one-fourth of all workers with back pain who don't get better, psychological and emotional factors are the key.

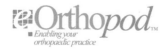

Notes

If you have similar concerns, talk them over with your doctor and therapist. Helping you overcome this fear is an important step in getting you safely back to work.

Researchers know that low back pain is often linked with anxiety or depression. The relationship is especially strong in patients whose pain doesn't get better. No one is exactly sure how this relationship works. Does the pain and inactivity cause anxiety and depression? Or does anxiety and depression set people up to have pain? The answer probably depends on the patient. But either way, it has become clear that doctors and therapists must deal with the psychological distress associated with low back pain in some patients.

A stressful job can deter a person from wanting to go back to work, especially for older workers. Older workers are particularly prone to the challenges a workplace can put on health. Stress can be a barrier for getting back to work, regardless of age. But for older workers especially, a stressful work setting makes back pain less tolerable and potentially more disabling. And older workers may be less free to change jobs to relieve the mental or emotional strain of work. Seek advice from your doctor and therapist about possible stresses at work that may be keeping you from wanting to go back to your job. If they don't have answers, they'll attempt to get you the help you need.

Join the Team

Everyone on the healthcare team is pulling for you. They want the best for you and your back. They'll help in every

Barriers to Getting Back to Work

- Older age
- Depression
- Poor fitness
- Heavy smoking
- Fear of re-injury
- Previous back injury
- Higher pain intensity
- Pending legal action
- Sciatica (leg pain coming from the back)

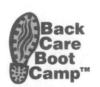

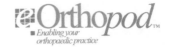

way to improve your safety at work (and play). You're on the team, too! What steps are you taking on your behalf? Are you applying the information and skills you've been learning in *Back Care Boot Camp*? If you smoke, have you taken steps to stop? If you are overweight, have you taken steps to lose weight? Are you trying to use safe posture, body mechanics, and lifting strategies? Have you discussed fears that may be keeping you from resuming normal daily and work activities?

You can also make a difference by taking note of your work tasks. How is your work or hobby environment arranged? Take a look at the items you must grasp, lift, and carry. Are they in a convenient spot? Or do you have to reach awkwardly to get them? Are the items bulky, heavy, or unpredictable? If you work long hours at a bench or in a chair you may need to be taught how to adjust them. If you have any questions or concerns about the safety of your work station or job tasks, let your therapist and doctor know. They'll work with others on the team to help you.

Skills to Master

You can take a role in managing your back condition at work or play. Develop healthy work practices by applying the skills listed below. The goal is to help you protect your back from future pain and problems. Not all choices are appropriate for everyone. Perform only the items recommended by your doctor or therapist.

Rearranging the Work Station

Ergonomics is the study of work and the work environment. The goal is to increase productivity by reducing fatigue and discomfort. Knowing how to rearrange a work station is important. We spend a large part of our lives at work. Efforts to improve our comfort at work and to make our work easier can pay off with reduced back strain.

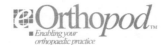
■ *Enabling your orthopaedic practice*

Adjusting Your Work Bench

Rationale

When you spend long hours at a work bench, your back may feel tired and sore. If so, it's possible that the height of the bench isn't adjusted properly. Back posture can be improved when your work bench is at just the right height.

Description

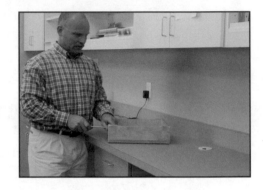

The best height for a typical work bench is where the top surface hits at your hip bone, just below your waistline. You can also check for proper height by standing in front of the work bench and noting the position of your back. Do you have to hunch forward as you work? If so, the surface is probably too low. If you work with small tools and objects, consider raising the surface so you can rest your elbows on the top of the bench as you work. Or sit with good back posture on a stool to get your hands in good position.

Recommendations

You may need to work with your therapist or supervisor to find ways to properly adjust the height of your work bench.

Concerns

Standing with awkward posture for long hours can take a toll on your back. Correcting the height of your work bench will help you keep your back in the neutral position. A low surface forces you to have to hunch over, which takes more energy than standing upright with good back posture.

Back Care Boot Camp™

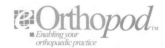

Orthopod™
Enabling your
orthopaedic practice

Adjusting Your Chair

Rationale

The position of your chair has a lot to do with the comfort of your back. An adjustable chair is ideal for getting your back aligned and supported in neutral.

Description

Ideally, you'll be able to choose an adjustable chair. Stand in front of the chair and adjust the chair up or down so the seat surface lines up with the bottom of your knee caps. Sit down, and check to see that there is at least 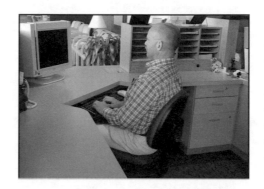 one finger's space between the seat and the backs of your knees. Next, adjust the lumbar support and chair back to fit snugly against the small of your back. Adjust the chair up or down until your feet are flat on the floor or a foot rest. Your thighs should be parallel to the floor. Angle the chair seat forward or backward for optimal support. If you have arm rests, adjust them for best comfort.

Recommendations

Adjusting your chair may not be enough. Training in how to adjust other office equipment, including the mouse, keyboard, and computer monitor, is equally important. Get assistance from your supervisor or therapist to properly align all parts of your workstation.

Concerns

Avoid slouching in the chair by keeping your low back firmly against the lumbar support. If your chair doesn't offer true lumbar support, roll up a towel or pillow to place in the small of the back. You could also purchase a commercial lumbar support to help keep your low back

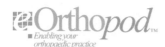

Notes

in its neutral position. Plan frequent breaks to get out of your chair to do some stretching, walking, and breathing.

Work Postures

Does your back feel tired and uncomfortable as the day goes on? Pay attention to your posture as you work. You've learned in previous sessions the importance of the neutral spine position. This is the ideal posture for the low back. You should strive for it when doing your work tasks. Whether you sit, stand, or walk as part of your job, paying attention to your work postures is a good starting point. It is a first step toward making adjustments to help you stay comfortable throughout your work day. Get in the habit of moving often to combat fatigue, discomfort, and pain.

Standing

Rationale

When you must stand for long periods, check your posture often. If you don't engage your trunk and hip muscles, you'll begin to rely on ligaments for postural support. The hips relax and begin to sag forward. The inward curve of the low back arches. The abdomen protrudes. Gravity pushes downward, putting a continuous strain on the spinal discs and ligaments. If you first align your back in its neutral posture while engaging your trunk muscles, your posture will be more efficient, and you'll avoid the fatigue and discomfort that comes with unhealthy standing postures.

Description

Place equal weight on both feet. Stand tall by lengthening your spine, elevating your ribs slightly and breath normally. Check your posture often to make sure you are keeping your low back in the neutral position.

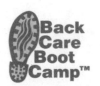

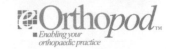
Enabling your orthopaedic practice

Recommendations

Your doctor or therapist may prescribe special insoles to reduce fatigue. People who stand in one place for long periods may benefit by standing on a commercial-type mat designed to reduce fatigue. Check your standing posture often. Correct your posture by "standing tall."

Concerns

Relying on your ligaments requires no effort, but it puts added strain on your low back. It takes a conscious and continual effort to stand in good posture and to use your trunk and hip muscles. Avoid relaxing into unhealthy standing postures.

Driving

Rationale

Driving is taxing on the low back. Driving is a risk factor for work-related back pain when people must drive more than half their workday. The vibration from the vehicle is one culprit. The other problem is that driving requires static sitting postures. High-mileage drivers must sit for long periods, which can produce discomfort and back soreness. Proper sitting postures can help, as can driving a vehicle with good seating. When possible, plan hourly breaks to get out, walk around, and do some stretching and breathing.

Description

The seat in your vehicle may not provide ideal sitting posture. Most seats are designed for the person of average height and weight, which means they fit few people well. You may need to experiment with commercial back and seating cushions. And

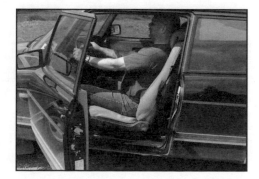

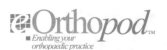

don't get stuck in one position. Routinely change positions by re-adjusting the seat or by applying or removing an optional back cushion. Use cruise control when it is safe. Stop at designated rest stops along your route. Get out. Go for a brisk walk, and do some stretching.

Recommendations

Your therapist may show you some stretches that can be done safely as you drive. You may be given a commercial back cushion or lumbar roll. Short drivers who end up driving with their legs straight forward may benefit by using pedal extensions. These extensions are typically available through the vehicle manufacturer. Follow the advice of your therapist and supervisor about taking rest breaks.

Concerns

High-mileage drivers are subject to back problems from vibration and from static sitting postures. The problem is compounded by poor seating. Drivers are advised to take breaks often, to get and stay in good shape, to avoid tobacco, and to monitor their body weight.

Taking Mini-Breaks

Rationale

The human body is made to move. Even staying too long in good posture can be harmful to the parts of the back. After about 15 minutes, supportive ligaments start to stretch out, and the discs and joints in the back become starved for the blood flow that normally comes with movement. Staying too long in one position also produces fatigue. Fatigue leads to discomfort and, eventually pain. The key is to upset this continuum by dealing with the hazards of fatigue—*before* they happen. Using mini-breaks gets the body moving and diminishes fatigue. This is also a way to stay alert and productive, while also improving work quality and safety.

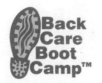

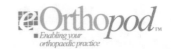

Description

Plan to stop and move
briefly every 15 to 20
minutes. Find other ways
to approach the task so
that your body gets a
break. For example, if
you've been standing at a

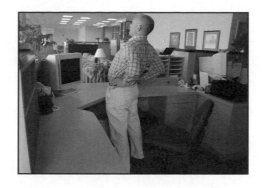

work bench, alternate by sitting on a stool. If you've been
bending over to work on a project, stop for a moment.
Stand up, place your hands on the small of your back,
and lean back for a slow and gentle stretch. Then resume
your task. People who are sitting for long periods can stop
and perform some movement right where they are. They
can reach their arms up toward the ceiling, bend back, or
stretch to the side. Plan a mini-break every 15 minutes so
you can pause, breathe, and move for 20 seconds or so.

Recommendations

Plan a mini-break every 15 to 20 minutes. Take a few
moments to relax, to breathe, and to do the stretches
demonstrated by your therapist.

Concerns

Don't get stuck in one position for too long. Plan ahead so
you can stop, move, and stretch. Feelings of fatigue and
discomfort are signals that something is wrong. If you
continue to work through them, you may be headed for
pain. Breaks to reduce muscle tension and fatigue must
be spaced throughout the day. Breathing and stretching
exercises should be an important part of the breaks.

Work Fitness

Have you noticed that when you feel good about your mind
and body, life and work are easy? That's where work fitness
comes in. It plays a significant role in reducing injuries at
work (and play). Promoting wellness and fitness are two

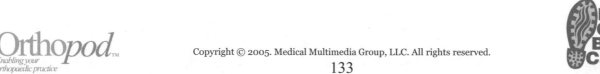

*Enabling your
orthopaedic practice*

Notes

important ways to keep life and work in proper perspective. The goal is to keep your body and back healthy.

Wellness

Rationale

You have some control over your spine health. One strategy for improved health and wellness is to know the risks for back problems and how to avoid them. Review the risks outlined earlier in this session. Which ones can you control? Attempt to deal with the risks within your control. Seek help when you need it. By taking action, you'll have an immediate impact on your quality of life and on the health of your back.

Description

Wellness is not the absence of disease. It's doing the best with what you've got. And it means taking action and making decisions to deal with problems. For instance, smoking is a known risk factor for back trouble. Taking steps to stop a nicotine habit is a major step toward improved wellness. Many resources are now available to help people who want to quit their habit.

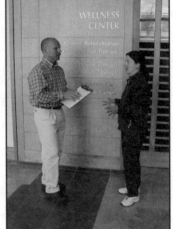

Other risks at work may need attention. You might need to work with your supervisor to control other parts of your job, such as the amount of overtime you are putting in. Outside resources are available to help with the ergonomics of your job, such as finding ways to improve your safety when dealing with heavy loads.

Recommendations

Seek out resources to help you improve your health and wellness. Start by discussing concerns with your doctor

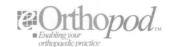

and therapist. They can work on your behalf to help you find a solution.

Concerns

Ignoring known risk factors is a roadblock to improved wellness. It's your back and your body. Improving wellness requires your involvement. It's your responsibility to make decisions and take actions to improve the health of your body and your back.

Physical Fitness

Rationale

People who are physically fit benefit from improved energy, alertness, and self-esteem. They are also generally better able to deal with stress, control body weight, and combat a variety of diseases.

Description

A well-rounded physical fitness program addresses flexibility, strength, aerobic conditioning, and relaxation.

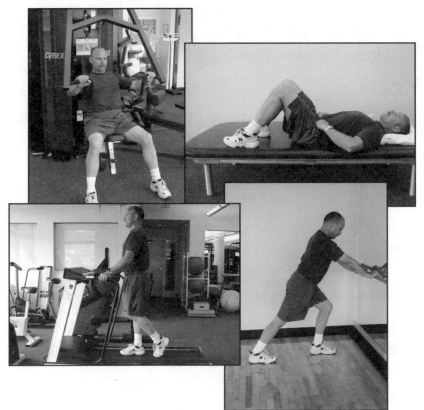

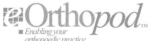
Enabling your orthopaedic practice

Back Care Boot Camp™

Notes

Examples of Moderate Activity

- Washing and waxing a car for 45-60 minutes
- Washing windows or floors for 45-60 minutes
- Playing volleyball for 45 minutes
- Playing touch football for 30-45 minutes
- Gardening for 30-45 minutes
- Wheeling yourself in a wheelchair for 30-40 minutes
- Playing wheelchair basketball for 20 minutes
- Playing basketball for 15-20 minutes
- Shooting baskets for 30 minutes

- Bicycling five miles in 30 minutes
- Fast dancing for 30 minutes
- Pushing a stroller 1.5 miles in 30 minutes
- Raking leaves for 30 minutes
- Walking two miles in 30 minutes
- Swimming laps for 20 minutes
- Bicycling four miles in 15 minutes
- Jumping rope for 15 minutes
- Running 1.5 miles in 15 minutes (10 min/mile)
- Shoveling snow for 15 minutes
- Walking stairs for 15 minutes

(From the Surgeon General's Report on Physical Activity and Health)

Recommendations

The Surgeon General recommends 30 minutes of moderate activity on most days of the week. (Refer to the box above for examples of moderate activity.)

Concerns

Being physically fit may not prevent a back problem. But people who stay active and who work on flexibility, strength, and endurance seem better able to manage back pain once it strikes. People who are sedentary and unfit are subject to back trouble, along with a host of preventable diseases such as colon cancer, joint problems, and heart disease.

Symptom Awareness

You can take an active role in heading off long-term back problems. Know the signs and symptoms that need attention.

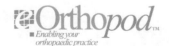

Report Problems Early

Rationale

By reporting problems early, you may be able to head off a major back problem. Too often, people rationalize their back pain by saying, "It'll go away in time." That's not always true. Sometimes, reporting the problem early will let your supervisor help you find solutions. Perhaps minor changes

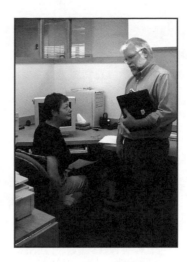

can be made in the way you do your job. Or maybe you need a checkup with your doctor or therapist. You'll get advice on what changes you can make to help you recover, and tips to keep the problem from happening again.

Description

Know these symptoms of back pain. They signal changes in your body that should act as a trigger for seeking help.

• Back discomfort that seems to be getting worse.

• Back pain that doesn't change when you rest or when you move around.

• New or increasing pain, numbness, or tingling in one or both legs.

• Changes in bowel or bladder function.

Recommendations

Talk to your supervisor, doctor, or therapist if you discover new back discomfort or pain.

Concerns

If you neglect the signals your body gives you, you may be headed for even bigger problems. If symptoms are left to linger, they may not go away. Worse yet, they may snowball. Get help early, rather than later. Solutions may be easier in the early days or weeks of a back problem, before they mount into a more challenging situation.

Special Situations

Shoveling

Rationale

It's hard to keep your back safely positioned while shoveling. You may have a tendency to twist and flex your back to get the job done. The key is to engage your core muscles and to generate power from your hip and leg muscles. Practicing good technique may seem awkward at first, but it helps by protecting your back during this work task.

Description

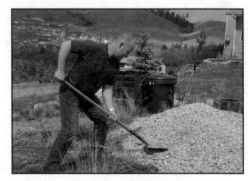

Approach the task head-on by facing the material you intend to shovel. Keep your back in the power position, and engage your core muscles. This will give you better leverage as you work the shovel. With each load, bend your hips and knees. As you move the material from one spot to another, avoid simply using your arms and twisting with your body. Instead, bend and move with your hips and knees so they do the work. You'll know you're shoveling safely if you keep your back in a straight line, with your hips directly behind you.

Recommendations

Practice engaging your core and using your arms and legs to shovel. People who do a lot of shoveling need extra strong hips and legs. Focus on the hips and legs in your strength and conditioning program.

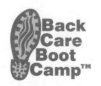
Back Care Boot Camp™

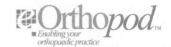
Orthopod™
Enabling your orthopaedic practice

Concerns

Avoid forcefully twisting sideways to heave the contents you are moving. If you don't engage your core muscles, you'll be forced to flex and twist your back. Remember to bend with your hips and knees rather than keeping your legs straight. Avoid hurling the contents with just your arms.

Care Giving

Taking care of other people is physically taxing. When the job requires lifting and moving people, the potential for back injuries goes way up. Reported back injuries among workers who have to move and lift other people, such as nurses, are staggering.

Rationale

Even with safe techniques and a strong back, lifting other people is a dangerous job. Some experts say that good technique and safe work practices are not enough. They recommend that moving and lifting people only be done with a mechanical lifting device. Even then, workers still must move and position the device safely. Other workers don't have a lifting device. They must be careful to use the body safely when lifting and moving people.

Description

If you don't have a lifting device, consider teaming up with a co-worker whenever possible to move and lift people. When you must work alone, be conscious about the position of your back at all times.

Check the List

Plan and prepare.

Use a wide base of support.

Keep the load close.

Use the neutral spine position.

Engage your core muscles.

Lift with your legs.

Avoid twisting.

Get help if needed.

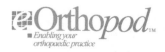

Notes

Apply the rules you learned in chapter four for safe lifting. The rules are listed for a quick refresher (see side bar). Along with safe lifting methods, always use a safety belt. The safety belt wraps around the person you intend to move. Apply the belt so it fits snuggly around the waist. Arrange the area for a smooth and safe transfer from one surface to the next. For example, if you're moving the individual from the bed to a chair, place the chair next to the bed to shorten the distance you need to go. Get as much help as possible from the person you are moving. Have her lean forward push off the bed with her hands. You can get extra leverage by holding the safety belt. Help her stand, turn, and then slowly sit in the chair.

Recommendations

Whenever possible, use a lifting device to lift and move others. If there is no lifting device work as a team. Only if necessary should you do the lift by yourself. Apply the concepts you've learned in *Back Care Boot Camp* to keep your back as safe as possible.

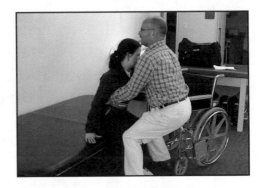

Concerns

Caring for others is a potential hazard for the back. More people report back pain in this industry than in jobs such as construction, logging, and factory work. When giving care to others, give some thought to caring for your back.

Self-Care

Taking care of your back involves taking care of yourself. With as many hours as you put in, consider yourself an industrial athlete. Think like an athlete. For instance,

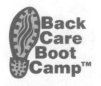

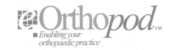

weight lifters do best when they give their bodies a rest after a heavy workout. By allowing their muscles time to recover, they get better results. They'll often work their chest and back muscles one day, and then do their legs or arms the next. Your body also needs a chance to renew after a hard day's work. Here are some ways to help you rest and recover.

- Apply a heating pad or cold pack on sore areas.

- Do some gentle stretches at lunch, during breaks, and after work.

- Take a brisk walk.

- Position your back comfortably and rest for 10 to 15 minutes.

- Engage the relaxation response.

Exercises

People who handle heavy items at work may think that's all the exercise they need. Others in less demanding jobs may conclude that only people in heavy jobs need to be in great shape. The truth is probably somewhere in between. When it comes to taking care of back problems, exercise has value. In Session Three you learned the importance of gaining strength and coordination of the core muscles. The same can be said about toning the muscles of the shoulders, arms, hips, and legs. You may not need a well-rounded strength and conditioning program in order to do your job better, but your back can sure benefit. As you near the end of *Back Care Boot Camp*, your therapist will put the finishing touches on an exercise program that you can enjoy for a lifetime.

Drill Time

Practice the skills and exercises shown by your therapist in this session. You'll be asked to demonstrate them during

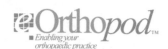
Enabling your orthopaedic practice

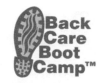
Back Care Boot Camp™

Notes

your next clinic visit. If you have pain or problems while practicing, your therapist can help at your next Drill Time.

Demonstrate

You may have been shown some or all of the items listed below. Go over them with your therapist to make sure you're doing them safely and correctly.

Engaging the Relaxation Response

- Breathing
- Relaxing
- Meditating
- Focusing

Making a Plan

- Identify ways to actively pursue lifelong spine health.
- Find programs and services in your location.
- Complete the form called *Making a Plan*.

Practice

Use this list as a reminder of the skills and exercises you'll be practicing. Practice only the skills and exercises shown by your therapist. Don't create your own exercises or go on to the next level without talking to your therapist.

Rearranging the Workstation

- Adjusting your work bench
- Adjusting your chair

Work Postures

- Standing
- Driving
- Taking mini-breaks

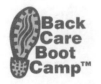

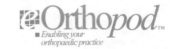

Notes

Work Fitness

- Wellness
- Physical fitness

Symptom Awareness

- Reporting problems early

Special Situations

- Shoveling
- Care giving

Self-Care

- Applying heat or cold
- Stretching
- Walking
- Positioning
- Relaxing

Exercises

- Core exercise
- Strength and conditioning exercise
- Aerobic exercise
- Home program

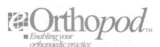

Notes

Questions for Review

1. How can fear keep a person from getting back to work?

2. How do you define ergonomics?

3. How do wellness and physical fitness improve spine health at work?

Think about these questions. They will be reviewed at the start of your next session.

Session Review

It is important that people with back pain return to work soon.

- The longer people stay off work, the greater their risk for long-term pain and disability.

- People at work tend to stay more active.

- They enjoy the social interaction of being at work.

- Their self-image is raised because they see themselves in a productive role.

- They sense that they are well, not ill.

- They find that their pain, though often annoying, is not disabling.

Back Care Boot Camp™

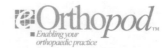
Enabling your
orthopaedic practice

The physical parts of a job contribute to work-related back pain.

- People who deal with heavy loads often report more back pain and back injuries.

- Lifting is often blamed as a cause of back pain, but lifting itself is not necessarily a risk factor until other variables are added.

- Vibration of the whole body is a risk factor for back pain.

- Driving can be a risk if people drive more than half the work day, probably because of static sitting posture and the vibration from the vehicle.

- Sedentary work is considered a risk factor for work-related back pain.

Workers' attitudes factor into work-related back pain.

- Having a sense of low job satisfaction.

- Feeling unable to influence work conditions.

- Working in a stressful work setting.

You take an active role in improving the ergonomics of your work (or hobby) environment.

- Make simple adjustments to work benches and chairs.

- Get additional training and help to improve the arrangement of the workstation.

- Take part in the company's work fitness program.

- Become more physically fit.

- Take mini-breaks often.

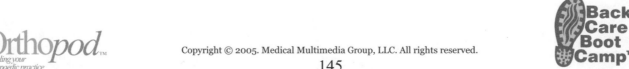
■ *Enabling your orthopaedic practice*

Notes

A well-rounded physical fitness program is important.

- It addresses flexibility, strength, aerobic conditioning, and relaxation.

- The Surgeon General recommends 30 minutes of moderate activity on most days of the week.

- People who stay active and who work on flexibility, strength, and endurance seem better able to manage back pain once it strikes.

- People who are sedentary and unfit are subject to back trouble, along with a host of preventable diseases such as colon cancer, joint problems, and heart disease.

Certain symptoms should be reported to your supervisor or doctor.

- Back discomfort that seems to be getting worse.

- Back pain that doesn't change when you rest or when you move around.

- Pain, numbness, or tingling in one or both legs.

- Back pain that happens during a specific work task.

- Changes in bowel or bladder function.

- Pain that awakens you in the middle of the night.

Back Care Boot Camp™

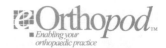
Enabling your orthopaedic practice

Session Eight: Back to the Future

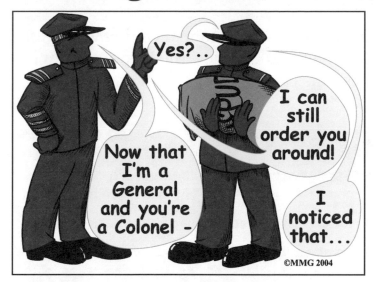

Goals for This Session

- Know what to do and where to go for lifelong spine health.

- Find enjoyable ways to keep your back fit and healthy.

- Define the idea behind *complementary medicine*.

- Create a plan to take care of your back for a lifetime.

- Demonstrate the skills you've learned in *Back Care Boot Camp*.

- Get your questions answered.

- Receive your certificate for completing *Back Care Boot Camp*.

Information to Master

This is your last session of *Back Care Boot Camp*. But it's your first step toward lifelong spine health. In this session, you'll be encouraged to get any last-minute questions answered. You'll also learn where to go and what to do next, which includes choosing an active routine to keep your back in tip-top shape. You'll also find there

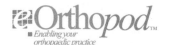

Notes

are other resources to complement what you've learned and done this far.

Before jumping ahead, spend time recalling what you learned in Session Seven. Review the answers from last session's Questions for Review.

Answers for Review

In the last session, you were asked three questions. Take a few moments to compare your answers to those given here.

1. How can fear keep a person from getting back to work?

People may be afraid that they'll hurt themselves again. Their fear may hold them back from being active, which can cause them to become unfit and even more aware of their pain. Their fear of re-injury strongly predicts that they'll have a harder time getting back to their jobs. Helping them overcome this fear is an important step in getting safely and swiftly back to work.

2. How do you define ergonomics?

It's the study of work and how to make it more efficient for each worker. The goal is to increase productivity by reducing fatigue and discomfort. It can include rearranging the workstation, modifying tools, taking rest breaks, and implementing work safety programs.

3. How do wellness and physical fitness improve spine health at work?

Wellness at work is all about action. It describes the worker who knows the risks for back problems and how to avoid them. It means taking action and making decisions to deal with problem areas. *Physical fitness* is important because it helps workers have improved energy, alertness, and self-esteem. It addresses flexibility, strength, aerobic conditioning, and relaxation. The Surgeon General reports that 30 minutes of activity on most days of the week improves physical fitness.

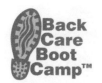

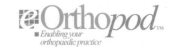

Notes

What's Next?

Your formal training in *Back Care Boot Camp* is nearly over. You've followed the syllabus step by step, done the exercises, and applied the tips you've learned. So where do you go from here?

Practice what you know. Check yourself often each day to ensure you're putting what you know to work. How's your posture? Is your back positioned safely when you sit, stand, and walk? Are you lifting with back safety in mind? Have you engaged your core muscles lately? The health of your spine depends on the actions you take to keep your back toned and safe. It's up to you to put into practice the ideas that can protect your back long into the future.

Manage your back condition. The goal of *Back Care Boot Camp* is to help you take control, to be self-sufficient in caring for your back. If your symptoms flare up—and likely they will—you've got the tools and know-how to manage them. You may need to back off for a short while. And then you'll gradually resume familiar activities and exercises. If you're having new and different symptoms, or if you're experiencing "red flag" symptoms (refer to Session Six), then see your doctor right away.

Refresh your spine know-how often. The course syllabus and accompanying information are yours to keep. Use them as a refresher. Challenge your knowledge by answering again the Questions for Review. Use the syllabus as a resource when you need to strategize a complex lifting situation or when you see a potential back hazard at work.

Do your exercises daily. You've learned a number of helpful exercises that are designed to improve your comfort and to protect your back for the years ahead. Don't quit doing them simply because you've completed your formal sessions. Unless your doctor or therapist instructs otherwise, continue doing the exercises you've

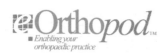

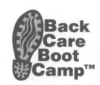

Notes

learned. Today's research shows that people who stay on a course of exercise fare best.

Find a favorite activity for the future. Along with keeping up on your exercises, find one or more enjoyable ways to stay active and motivated in taking care of your back. Do you love to swim? Then find a program where you can join others who swim. Do you enjoy exercising at a gym? Get a membership and begin working out at a nearby fitness club. You don't have to join a specialized program to stay active. A personalized exercise program may be right for you. Perhaps you'd prefer more of a mind-body way to keep your back healthy. Try yoga or Tai Chi. Seeking to maximize your core strength? Pursue individual or group Pilates exercise.

Finding the Right Routine

- Aquatics
- Fitness
- Personalized exercise
- Pilates
- Tai Chi
- Yoga

Choose Your Future

As you look to the future, it is crucial to find activities that you like. It's easy to stick with a program that you really enjoy. The key is to choose an active routine, rather than passive treatment.

Aquatics

Exercising in a pool is a great way to keep your back healthy for the years ahead. Working in the water puts less stress on the low back than exercising on land. The warm water helps relax muscles, and the buoyancy allows for easier movement during exercise. Many health clubs offer pool memberships. Some have group exercises for the spine.

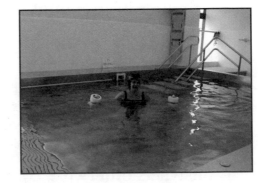

Back Care Boot Camp™

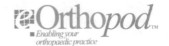
Orthopod™
■ Enabling your orthopaedic practice

Fitness

People who have had back pain benefit by staying fit. Joining a health club may be a way for you to keep up with an active routine. Many health clubs run classes and group programs to improve core strengthening, aerobic conditioning, and flexibility. Your therapist can work with trainers at the fitness facility to design a program that's right for you.

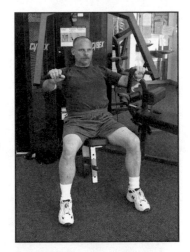

Personalized Exercise

There are many active exercise routines you can do on your own. Start with the home program demonstrated by your therapist. This routine may be all that you need to keep your back flexible and strong. You may wish to supplement your individual program by purchasing exercise equipment, videos, or books. Take steps throughout the day to increase your activity for added fitness benefits.

Get Moving

- Take the stairs, not the elevator.

- Park further away to increase your walk to work or the store.

- Take a brisk walk instead of eating a snack.

- Rake your own leaves.

- Mow your own lawn.

- Pick up the pace when working in the house or yard.

- Take mini-breaks during work hours to stretch and walk.

- Carry your own groceries.

Pilates

The Pilates method of body conditioning has been used successfully by dancers for many years. It is one of the fastest growing exercise programs today, benefiting people of all ages and activity levels. Pilates provides a well-rounded fitness program which focuses on core stabilization. The exercises simultaneously stretch,

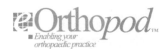

Notes

strengthen, and align the body. Pilates emphasizes resistance during movement, which requires precisely controlled actions of the body's inner muscles. Pilates promotes the mind-body connection by repeating various exercises, producing lasting change in posture, body balance, and core stability.

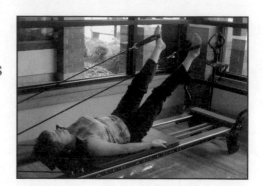

Tai Chi

Originating in China in the 1300s, Tai Chi is now a popular form of exercise in the West. It is based on the circulation of energy (qigong), which provides self-healing through movement. It is well suited for people with back pain because it teaches you to become aware of your posture and movement. The various forms of Tai Chi integrate your mind and body. The movements are gentle, yet they foster improved flexibility, coordination, balance, and strength.

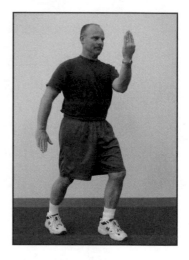

Yoga

Yoga is a 5,000-year-old system. It developed in India and provides a complete philosophy of living. The word *yoga* means "to yoke or join together." Yoga unites the mind and body through specific poses and breath work.

Yoga can help mend the back and keep your back healthy. Practicing yoga creates strength, flexibility, improved posture, and body awareness. Breath work and relaxation help to ease tension and stress.

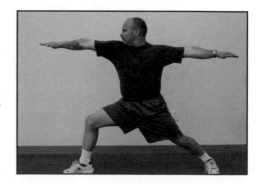

Back Care Boot Camp™

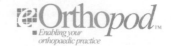
Orthopod™
■ *Enabling your orthopaedic practice*

Pay a "Complement" to Other Healthcare Providers

Where do people get help when they have back pain? Most people see their doctor. They may also get help from other types of healthcare services. These other services can complement traditional medical help. Chiropractic care, massage, and herbal medicine are examples of *complementary and alternative medicine* (CAM) therapies.

CAM is built on the idea that our bodies can self-heal. CAM practitioners look at the whole person. They treat the mind, body, and occasionally the spirit in order to foster inner healing of the body.

Twenty-five percent of back and neck pain patients combine medical care along with CAM therapies. Some people find improved results in preventing and treating illness, disease, and pain. The two forms of care must be coordinated for the best results.

As you complete your journey through *Back Care Boot Camp*, know that you are in charge of your spine health. You must make the connection between your current and future health. Many options and choices are in vogue and can help cinch this connection. Your next step is to complete your strategy for lifelong spine health.

Skills to Master

Congratulations! You've mastered a set of skills that can help you take care of your back for the years ahead. In this wrap-up session, you'll take the steps needed to finish your plan for the future. There are lots of ways you can stay active and keep your back healthy. By now you should know the strategy you'll use to help you achieve lifelong spine health.

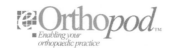

Notes

Skills Review

You've had back pain once. You can almost bet you'll have it again sometime in the future. As you now know, nine out of 10 people who've had it once will have back pain again. The key is to know what to do for it when it happens. Each skill you've learned in *Back Care Boot Camp* can help you take care of your back for the years ahead. Take a moment now to review all the skills you learned in previous lessons. Work with your physical therapist to make sure you're doing them correctly.

Self-care	remedies	positioning	movements	management
Posture	sitting	standing	driving	computing
Core stability	muscle activation	abdominal bracing	sit to stand	hinged squat
Body mechanics	sitting & standing	sweeping	mopping	vacuuming
Lifting	golfer's lift	diagonal lift	power lift	situations
Aerobic exercise	activity choices	calculating intensity	duration	intensity
Exercise	pelvic tilt	cat & camel	stretching	home program
Relaxation	breathing	relaxing	meditating	focusing

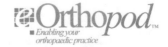

Notes

Drill Time

Continue to practice the skills and exercises that you've learned in *Back Care Boot Camp*. If you have pain or problems while practicing, notify your therapist.

Demonstrate

You may have been shown some or all of the items listed below. Go over them with your therapist to make sure you're doing them safely and correctly.

Rearranging Your Workstation

- Adjusting your work bench
- Adjusting your chair

Work Postures

- Standing
- Driving
- Taking mini-breaks

Work Fitness

- Wellness
- Physical fitness

Symptom Awareness

- Early reporting

Special Situations

- Shoveling
- Care giving

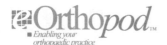

Notes

Self-Care

- Applying heat or cold
- Stretching
- Walking
- Positioning
- Relaxing

Exercise

- Core exercise
- Strength and conditioning exercise
- Aerobic exercise
- Home program

Questions for Review

1. In what ways are you self-sufficient in taking care of your back?

2. Which resources are available and appeal to you the most?

3. How do you plan to actively improve your spine health for the future?

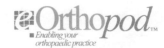

Notes

Session Review

Congratulations. You've completed *Back Care Boot Camp.*

- Practice what you know.

- Manage the best you can.

- Refresh your spine know-how often.

- Do your exercises daily.

- Find a favorite activity to promote lifelong spine health.

Find an active routine that's right for you.

- Aquatics

- Fitness

- Personalized exercise

- Pilates

- Tai Chi

- Yoga

Complementary and alternative medical therapies are available.

- CAM treatments include chiropractic care, massage, and herbal medicine.

- CAM is built on the idea that our bodies can self-heal.

- CAM practitioners treat the mind, body, and occasionally the spirit.

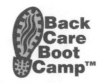

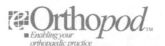

Notes

Take care of your spine for the future.

- Form a plan to follow an active routine.

- Apply the principles you've learned in *Back Care Boot Camp*.

- Continually make spine-healthy decisions about daily habits, postures, lifting safety, and self-care.

Congratulations!

You completed *Back Care Boot Camp*. Upon submitting your completed plan to your therapist, you are entitled to receive your graduation certificate. Cheers to you and to the future health of your back!

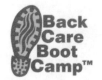

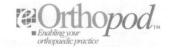

Making a Plan

Use this form to help establish your future plan.

By completing this form, you are developing a strategy to help you achieve lifelong spine health. When you've made a plan, go over it with your healthcare provider.

Consider these options.

Refer to Session Eight for more information on the options listed here. This is just a starting point of the many programs and possibilities that are now available to help people achieve optimal spine health.

1. Aquatics
2. Fitness
3. Personal exercise
4. Pilates
5. Tai Chi
6. Yoga

Check these sources.

Find programs and services in your location using these and other sources.

1. Newspaper
2. Phone book
3. Health club bulletin boards
4. Internet

Here is my plan.

I've created a strategy for lifelong spine health that includes

_____

_____

_____

_____

_____   _____
Participant   Healthcare Provider

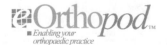

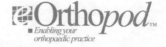

Patient Specific Functional Scale

Name: _____ Date: _____

Identify three important activities that you are unable to do or have difficulty with as a result of your problem. List each activity in the left column of the box below.

Today, how difficult is it to perform each activity?

Chose a number between zero and 10 indicating your ability to do each activity. Place your number in the score column in the box below to the right of the activity you've listed.

| 0 | 1 | 2 | 3 | 4 | 5 | 6 | 7 | 8 | 9 | 10 |

unable to
perform activity

able to perform activity
at preinjury level

Activity	Score
1.	
2.	
3.	

Raw score _____ **Percentage (raw score/30 x 100)** _____

Source

Reprinted from *Physiotherapy Canada*. Vol. 47. Paul W. Stratford, PT, MSc, et al. Assessing Disability and Change on Individual Patients: A Report of a Patient Specific Measure. Pp. 258-263. © Stratford, 1995, reprinted with permission.

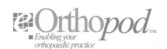

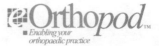

Oswestry Disability Index

Name: _____ Date: _____

The questionnaire is designed to give us information as to how your back (or leg) trouble has affected your ability to manage in everyday life. Please answer every section. Mark one box only in each section that most closely describes you today.

Section 1 - Pain Intensity

____ I have no pain at the moment.

____ The pain is very mild at the moment.

____ The pain is moderate at the moment.

____ The pain is fairly severe at the moment.

____ The pain is very severe at the moment.

____ The pain is the worst imaginable at the moment.

Section 2 - Personal Care (washing, dressing, etc.)

____ I can look after myself normally without causing extra pain.

____ I can look after myself normally but it is very painful.

____ It is painful to look after myself and I am slow and careful.

____ I need some help but manage most of my personal care.

____ I need help every day in most aspects of self care.

____ I do not get dressed, wash with difficulty and stay in bed.

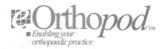

Section 3 - Lifting

____ I can lift heavy weights without extra pain.

____ I can lift heavy weights but it gives extra pain.

____ Pain prevents me from lifting heavy weights off the floor but I can manage if they are conveniently positioned, e.g. on a table.

____ Pain prevents me from lifting heavy weights but I can manage light to medium weights if they are conveniently positioned.

____ I can lift only very light weights.

____ I cannot lift or carry anything at all.

Section 4 - Walking

____ Pain does not prevent me walking any distance.

____ Pain prevents me walking more than one mile.

____ Pain prevents me walking more than a quarter of a mile.

____ Pain prevents me walking more than 100 yards.

____ I can only walk using a stick or crutches.

____ I am in bed most of the time and have to crawl to the toilet.

Section 5 - Sitting

____ I can sit in any chair as long as I like.

____ I can sit in my favorite chair as long as I like.

____ Pain prevents me from sitting for more than 1 hour.

____ Pain prevents me from sitting for more than half an hour.

____ Pain prevents me from sitting for more than 10 minutes.

____ Pain prevents me from sitting at all.

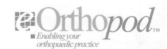

Section 6 - Standing

_____ I can stand as long as I want without extra pain.

_____ I can stand as long as I want but it gives me extra pain.

_____ Pain prevents me from standing for more than 1 hour.

_____ Pain prevents me from standing for more than half an hour.

_____ Pain prevents me from standing for more than 10 minutes.

_____ Pain prevents me from standing at all.

Section 7 - Sleeping

_____ My sleep is never disturbed by pain.

_____ My sleep is occasionally disturbed by pain.

_____ Because of pain I have less than 6 hours sleep.

_____ Because of pain I have less than 4 hours sleep.

_____ Because of pain I have less than 2 hours sleep.

_____ Pain prevents me from sleeping at all.

Section 8 - Sex Life (if applicable)

_____ My sex life is normal and causes no extra pain.

_____ My sex life is normal but causes some extra pain.

_____ My sex life is normal but is very painful.

_____ My sex life is severely restricted by pain.

_____ My sex life is nearly absent because of pain.

_____ Pain prevents any sex life at all.

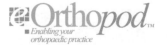

Section 9 - Social Life

_____ My social life is normal and causes me no extra pain.

_____ My social life is normal but increases the degree of pain.

_____ Pain has no significant effect on my social life apart from limiting my more energetic interests, e.g. sport, etc.

_____ Pain has restricted my social life and I do not go out as often.

_____ Pain has restricted social life to my home.

_____ I have no social life because of pain.

Section 10 - Traveling

_____ I can travel anywhere without pain.

_____ I can travel anywhere but it gives extra pain.

_____ Pain is bad but I manage journeys over two hours.

_____ Pain restricts me to journeys of less than one hour.

_____ Pain restricts me to short necessary journeys under 30 minutes.

_____ Pain prevents me from traveling except to receive treatment.

Raw score _____ **Percentage (total score/total possible x 100)** _____

Level of disability _____

Source

Reprinted from _Physiotherapy_. Vol. 66. J Fairbank, et al. The Oswestry Disability Index V2.1. Pp. 271–273. © 1983, with permission from Jeremy Fairbank, MD, FRCS.

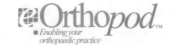

Visual Analog Scale

Name: _____ Date : _____

Place a vertical mark on the line below to indicate your present pain level.

_____

No symptoms   Severe symptoms

Source

Reprinted from *Pain*. Vol. 16. A. M. Carlsson. Assessment of Chronic Pain: Aspects of the Reliability and Validity of the Visual Analog Scale. Pp. 87–101. © 1983, with permission from The International Association for the Study of Pain.

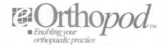

167

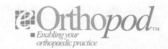

Fear-Avoidance Beliefs Questionnaire

Name: _____ Date: _____

Here are some of the things other patients have told us about their pain. For each statement, please circle the number from 0 to 6 to indicate how much physical activities such as bending, lifting, walking, or driving affect or would affect your back pain.

	Completely Disagree			Unsure			Completely Agree
1. My pain was caused by physical activity.	0	1	2	3	4	5	6
2. Physical activity makes my pain worse.	0	1	2	3	4	5	6
3. Physical activity might harm my back.	0	1	2	3	4	5	6
4. I should not do physical activities which (might) make my pain worse.	0	1	2	3	4	5	6
5. I cannot do physical activities which (might) make my pain worse.	0	1	2	3	4	5	6

Physical activity subscale (numbers 2, 3, 4, & 5) = _____

The following statements are about how your normal work affects or would affect your back pain.

	Completely Disagree			Unsure			Completely Agree
6. My pain was caused by my work or by an accident at work.	0	1	2	3	4	5	6

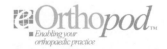

	Completely Disagree			Unsure		Completely Agree	
7. My work aggravated my pain.	0	1	2	3	4	5	6
8. I have a claim for compensation for my pain.	0	1	2	3	4	5	6
9. My work is too heavy for me.	0	1	2	3	4	5	6
10. My work makes or would make my pain worse.	0	1	2	3	4	5	6
11. My work might harm my back.	0	1	2	3	4	5	6
12. I should not do my regular work with my present pain.	0	1	2	3	4	5	6
13. I cannot do my normal work with my present pain.	0	1	2	3	4	5	6
14. I cannot do my normal work until my pain is treated.	0	1	2	3	4	5	6
15. I do not think that I will be back to my normal work within 3 months.	0	1	2	3	4	5	6
16. I do not think that I will ever be able to go back to that work.	0	1	2	3	4	5	6

Work subscale = (numbers 6, 7, 9, 10, 11, 12, & 15) = _____

Total raw score (numbers 1 – 16) = _____

Source

Reprinted from *Pain*. Vol. 52. G Waddell, et al. A Fear-Avoidance Beliefs Questionnaire (FABQ) and the Role of Fear-Avoidance in Chronic Low Back Pain and Disability. Pp. 157–168. © 1993, with permission from The International Association for the Study of Pain.

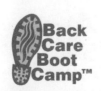

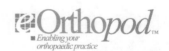

Scoring the Patient Specific Functional Scale

Instructions

Read the instructions (provided below) to the patient. Fill in the patient's answers in the box accompanying the functional scale.

Read at baseline assessment

I'm going to ask you to identify three important activities that you are unable to do or have difficulty with as a result of your problem. Today, how difficult is it to perform activity 1 (have patient score this activity); 2 (have patient score this activity); 3 (have patient score this activity).

Read at follow up assessment

When I assessed you on (state previous assessment date), you told me that you had difficulty performing these activities (read 1, 2, 3 from list). Today do you still have difficulty with activity 1 (have patient score this activity); 2 (have patient score this activity); 3 (have patient score this activity).

Scoring Interpretation

Using the baseline activities listed by the patient, compare scores at routine intervals (every two to four weeks) to track changes. Calculate the raw score by adding the total scores of the three activities. You can also track the score as a percentage (by dividing the total score by 30 and then multiplying by 100). Correlate changes in the patient's scores with clinical measures and with scales of physical impairment (e.g. Oswestry Disability Index).

Scoring Significance

The patient specific functional scale (PSFS) is highly responsive, meaning it can detect clinically significant changes in a patient's health. Physical impairment measures are not as helpful for showing change with treatment. Thus, improvements in the PSFS scores are good indicators that the patient is benefiting from a functional standpoint with the treatment.

Source

Reprinted from *Physiotherapy Canada*. Vol. 47. Paul W. Stratford, PT, MSc, et al. Assessing Disability and Change on Individual Patients: A Report of a Patient Specific Measure. Pp. 258-263. © Stratford, 1995, reprinted with permission.

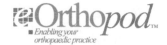

Back Care Boot Camp™

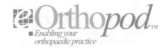

Scoring the Oswestry Disability Index

Scoring Examples

Score: / x 100 = %

For each section, the total possible score is five. If the first answer is marked, the score is zero. If the last answer is marked, the score is five.
If all ten categories are marked, the score is calculated as follows:

Example: 16 (total scored)
            50 (total possible score) x 100 = 32%

If one category is missed or not applicable, the score is calculated as follows:

Example: 16 (total scored)
            45 (total possible score) x 100 = 35.6%

(For convenience, round the percentage to a whole number.)

Score Interpretation

0% to 20%: minimal disability

21% to 40%: moderate disability

41% to 60%: severe disability

61% to 80%: crippled

81% to 100%: bed-bound or exaggerating

Score Significance

The minimal detectable change can be noted with 90% confidence. A change of less than 10% may be attributable to an error in measurement.

Source

Reprinted from *Physiotherapy*. Vol. 66. J Fairbank, et al. The Oswestry Disability Index V2.1. Pp. 271–273. © 1983, with permission from Jeremy Fairbank, MD, FRCS.

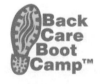

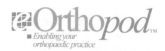

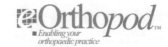

Scoring the Fear-Avoidance Beliefs Questionnaire

Summing Items

Each item is scored zero to six, with higher numbers indicating increased levels of fear-avoidance beliefs. Two subscales are included in the questionnaire. The first is a four-item physical activity subscale (green numbers 2, 3, 4, & 5) with a score range of zero to 24. The second is a seven-item work subscale (brown numbers 6, 7, 9, 10, 11, 12, & 15) with a score range of zero to 42. Add up the scores in each subscale and for the entire questionnaire. The maximum possible score for the fear-avoidance beliefs questionnaire is 96. The raw scores are usually reported, not percentages.

Significance

Elevated fear-avoidance beliefs are not indicative of a "red flag" (i.e. serious medical pathology). Instead, they are indicative of someone who has a poorer prognosis. As such, they are more accurately labeled a "yellow flag" (indicating psychosocial involvement). Elevated fear-avoidance beliefs suggest that the clinician change the management approach and include education that addresses the patient's fear and avoidance behavior. Also, consider a graded approach to therapeutic exercise, one that gradually increases the exercise prescription (frequency, intensity, and duration). In this model, focus is on the amount of exercise performed and not on the presence of symptoms.

Physical Activity Scores

Scores above 14 in the physical activity scale are considered "high" and may suggest that the patient is likely to be an "avoider." If a person has a score of 14 or more, this does not necessarily mean there is an increased chance of prolonged disability. When comparing outcome scores in the physical activity subscale, changes equal to or greater than four are considered clinically important.

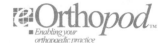

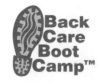

Work Scores

Researchers have found an association between work-scale scores and whether patients get back to work. People with work-scale scores over 34 have an increased risk of not returning to work. Work-scale scores less than 29 indicate a decreased risk of not returning to work.

Source

Reprinted from *Pain*. Vol. 52. G Waddell, et al. A Fear-Avoidance Beliefs Questionnaire (FABQ) and the Role of Fear-Avoidance in Chronic Low Back Pain and Disability. Pp. 157–168. © 1993, with permission from The International Association for the Study of Pain.

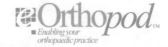

Progress Flow Chart

Patient: _____ Doctor: _____

Session Completion

Keep track of the dates in which the following sessions are completed.

Session	Date Completed	Comments
Back in Action		
Take Your Position		
Hold Steady		
Ready, Set, Lift!		
Back Pain Basics		
Mastering Your Back Pain		
Back to Work		
Back to the Future		

Outcomes Tracking

Keep track of the outcomes scores from baseline to discharge. Calculate the scores, either as a percentage or as a "raw" score, using the total values (supplied in parentheses).

Outcomes Measures	Baseline Date/Score	Interim Date/Score	Interim Date/Score	Discharge Date/Score
Patient Specific Functional Scale (30)				
Oswestry Disability Index (50)				
Visual Analogue Scale (10)				
Fear-Avoidance Beliefs Questionnaire (96)				

Comments

_____

_____

_____

_____

Physical Therapist

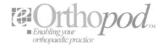

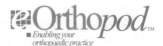

CERTIFICATE OF ACHIEVEMENT

BACK CARE BOOT CAMP™

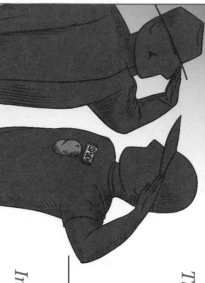

This certificate is presented to

In recognition of successfully completing
Back Care Boot Camp™

Signature

Date

Signature

Date

References

Active Rehabilitation

Steven Z. George, MS, PT, et al. A Comparison of Fear-Avoidance Beliefs in Patients with Lumbar Spine Pain and Cervical Spine Pain. In *Spine*. October 1, 2001. Vol. 26. No. 19. Pp. 2139-2145.

Eli Molde Hagen, MD, et al. Does Early Intervention with a Light Mobilization Program Reduce Long-Term Sick Leave for Low Back Pain. In *Spine*. August 1, 2000. Vol. 25. No. 15. Pp. 1973-1976.

Anne F. Mannion, PhD, et al. Active Therapy for Chronic Low Back Pain: Part 3. Factors Influencing Self-Rated Disability and Its Change Following Therapy. In *Spine*. April 15, 2001. Vol. 26. No. 8. Pp. 920-929.

Sylvie Rozenberg, MD, et al. Bed Rest or Normal Activity for Patients with Acute Low Back Pain. In *Spine*. July 15, 2002. Vol. 27. No. 14. Pp. 1487-1493.

Inger B. Scheel, DC, MOH, et al. A Call for Action: A Randomized Controlled Trial of Two Strategies to Implement Active Sick Leave for Patients with Low Back Pain. In *Spine*. March 15, 2002. Vol. 27. No. 6. Pp. 561-566.

Maurits W. van Tulder, PhD, and Gordon Waddell, DSc, MD, FRCS. Conservative Treatment of Acute and Subacute Low Back Pain. *Neck and Back Pain: The Scientific Evidence of Causes, Diagnosis, and Treatment*. Eds Alf L. Nachemson, MD, PhD, and Egon Jonsson, PhD. Lipincott, Williams, & Wilkins. Philadelphia, PA. 2000. Pp. 241-269.

Complementary Medicine

Peter M. Wolsko, MD, MPH, et al. Patterns and Perceptions of Care for Treatment of Back and Neck Pain: Results of a National Survey. In *Spine*. January 1, 2003. Vol. 28. No. 3. Pp. 292-298.

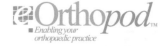
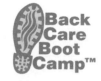

Ergonomics

Benjamin C. Amick III, PhD, et al. Effect of Office Ergonomics Intervention on Reducing Musculoskeletal Symptoms. In *Spine*. December 15, 2003. Vol. 28. No. 24. Pp. 2706-2711.

Lifting

Wilhelmina E. Hoogendoorn, MSc, et al. Flexion and Rotation of the Trunk and Lifting at Work are Risk Factors for Low Back Pain: Results of a Prospective Cohort Study. In *Spine*. December 15, 2000. Vol. 25. No. 23. Pp. 3087-3092.

Yung-Hui Lee, PhD, and Tzu-Hsien Lee, MS. Human Muscular and Postural Responses in Unstable Load Lifting. In *Spine*. September 1, 2002. Vol. 27. No. 17. Pp. 1881-1886.

William S. Marras, PhD, et al. Spine Loading Characteristics of Patients with Low Back Pain Compared with Asymptomatic Individuals. In *Spine*. December 1, 2001. Vol. 26. No. 23. Pp. 2566-2574.

Joan M. Stevenson, PhD, et al. A Longitudinal Study of the Development of Low Back Pain in an Industrial Population. In *Spine*. June 15, 2001. Vol. 26. No. 12. Pp. 1370-1377.

J. (Petra) C. E. van der Burg, MSc, et al. Effects of Unexpected Lateral Mass Placement on Trunk Loading in Lifting. In *Spine*. April 15, 2003. Vol. 28. No. 8. Pp. 764-770.

Simon S. Yeung, MPhil, PT, et al. Prevalence of Musculoskeletal Symptoms in Single and Multiple Body Regions and Effects of Perceived Risk of Injury among Manual Handling Workers. In *Spine*. October 1, 2002. Vol. 27. No. 19. Pp. 2166-2172.

Lumbar Stabilization

Jacek Cholewicki, PhD, et al. Neuromuscular Function in Athletes Following Recovery from a Recent Acute Low Back Injury. In *Journal of Orthopaedic & Sports Physical Therapy*. November 2002. Vol. 32. No. 11. Pp. 568-575.

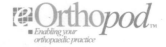

Carolyn Richardson, PhD, BPhty (Hons), et al. *Therapeutic Exercise for Spinal Segmental Stabilization in Low Back Pain: Scientific Basis and Clinical Approach*. Churchill Livingstone. Philadelphia, PA. 1999.

Obesity and Back Pain

Jason C. Fanuele, MS, et al. Association between Obesity and Functional Status in Patients with Spine Disease. In *Spine*. February 1, 2002. Vol. 27. No. 3. Pp. 306-312.

Posture

Gerold R. Ebenbichler, et al. Sensory-Motor Control of the Lower Back: Implications for Rehabilitation. In *Medicine & Science in Sports & Exercise*. November 2001. Vol. 33. No. 11. Pp. 1889-1898.

McLean Jackson, BSc, et al. Multifidus EMG and Tension-Relaxation Recovery after Prolonged Static Lumbar Flexion. In *Spine*. April 1, 2001. Vol. 26. No. 7. Pp. 715-723.

Proprioception

Peter B. O'Sullivan, PhD, et al. Lumbar Repositioning Deficit in a Specific Low Back Pain Population. In *Spine*. May 15, 2003. Vol. 28. No. 10. Pp. 1074-1079.

Questionnaires

A. M. Carlsson. Assessment of Chronic Pain: Aspects of the Reliability and Validity of the Visual Analog Scale. In *Pain*. 1983. Vol. 16. Pp. 87-101.

Megan Davidson, PT, BAppSc, and Jennifer L. Keating, PT, PhD. A Comparison of Five Low Back Disability Questionnaires: Reliability and Responsiveness. In *Physical Therapy*. January 2002. Vol. 82. No. 1. Pp. 8-24.

Jeremy Fairbank, MD, FRCS, et al. The Oswestry Disability Index V2.1. In *Physiotherapy*. 1983. Vol. 66. Pp. 271-273.

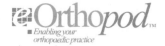

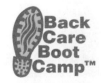

Julie M. Fritz, PT, ATC, and Sara R. Piva, MS, PT. Physical Impairment Index: Reliability, Validity, and Responsiveness in Patients with Acute Low Back Pain. In *Spine*. June 1, 2003. Vol. 28. No. 11. Pp. 1189-1194.

Steven Z. George, PT, PhD, et al. Physical Therapist Management of a Patient with Acute Low Back Pain and Elevated Fear-Avoidance Beliefs. In *Physical Therapy*. June 2004. Vol. 84. No. 6. Pp. 538-549.

Liset H. M. Pengel, MSc, et al. Responsiveness of Pain, Disability, and Physical Impairment Outcomes in Patients with Low Back Pain. In *Spine*. April 15, 2004. Vol. 29. No. 8. Pp. 879-883.

Paul W. Stratford, PT, MSc, et al. Assessing Disability and Change on Individual Patients: A Report of a Patient Specific Measure. In *Physiotherapy Canada*. 1995. Vol. 47. Pp. 258-263.

Gordon Waddell, DSc, MD, FRCS, et al. A Fear-Avoidance Beliefs Questionnaire (FABQ) and the Role of Fear-Avoidance Beliefs in Chronic Low Back Pain and Disability. In *Pain*. February 1993. Vol. 52. No. 2. Pp. 157-168.

Smoking and Back Pain

Anna-Lisa Hellsing, MMed, MSc, and Ing-Liss Bryngelsson. Predictors of Musculoskeletal Pain in Men: A Twenty-Year Follow-Up from Examination at Enlistment. In *Spine*. December 1, 2000. Vol. 35. No. 23. Pp. 3080-3086.

Glenn R. Rechtine II, MD, et al. Effect of the Spine Practitioner on Patient Smoking Status. In *Spine*. September 1, 2000. Vol. 25. No. 17. Pp. 2229-2233.

Molly T. Vogt, PhD, et al. Influence of Smoking on the Health Status of Spinal Patients. In *Spine*. February 1, 2002. Vol. 27. No. 3. Pp. 313-319.

Work-Injury Management

Rachelle Buchbinder, MBBS (Hons), MSc, FRACP, et al. 2001 Volvo Award Winner in Clinical Studies: Effects of a Media Campaign on Back Pain Beliefs and Its Potential Influence on Management of Low Back Pain in General Practice. In *Spine*. December 1, 2001. Vol. 26. No. 23. Pp. 2535-2542.

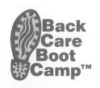

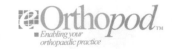

Marlene Fransen, PhD, et al. Risk Factors Associated with the Transition from Acute to Chronic Occupational Back Pain. In *Spine*. January 1, 2002. Vol. 27. No. 1. Pp. 92-98.

Julie M. Fritz, PT, PhD, ATC, and Steven Z. George, PT, MS. Identifying Psychosocial Variables in Patients with Acute Work-Related Low Back Pain: The Importance of Fear-Avoidance Beliefs. In *Physical Therapy*. October 2002. Vol. 82. No. 10. Pp. 973-983.

Steven Z. George, PT, PhD, et al. The Effect of a Fear-Avoidance-Based Physical Therapy Intervention for Patients with Acute Low Back Pain: Results of a Randomized Clinical Trial. In *Spine*. December 1, 2003. Vol. 28. No. 23. pp. 2551-2560.

Nortin M. Hadler, MD. Editorial: The Bane of the Aging Worker. In *Spine*. June 15, 2001. Vol. 26. No. 12. Pp. 1309-1310.

Rudi Hiebert, BS, et al. Work Restrictions and Outcome of Nonspecific Low Back Pain. In *Spine*. April 1, 2003. Vol. 28. No. 7. Pp. 722-728.

Kaija Karjalainen, MD, et al. Outcome Determinants of Subacute Low Back Pain. In *Spine*. December 1, 2003. Vol. 28. No. 23. Pp. 2634-2640.

K. A. Parks, BSc, et al. A Comparison of Lumbar Range of Motion and Functional Ability Scores in Patients with Low Back Pain. In *Spine*. February 15, 2003. Vol. 28. No. 4. Pp. 380-384.

Carina Thorbjornsson, M Soc Sc, et al. Physical and Psychosocial Factors Related to Low Back Pain during a 24-Year Period. In *Spine*. February 1, 2000. Vol. 25. No. 3. Pp. 369-375.

Gordon Waddell, DSc, MD, FRCS. *The Back Pain Revolution*. Churchill Livingston. Philadelphia, PA. 1998.

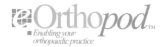

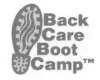

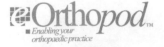